FEELING MEDICINE

BIOPOLITICS: MEDICINE, TECHNOSCIENCE, AND HEALTH IN THE TWENTY-FIRST CENTURY SERIES

General Editors: Monica J. Casper and Lisa Jean Moore

Feeling Medicine

How the Pelvic Exam Shapes Medical Training

Kelly Underman

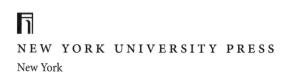

NEW YORK UNIVERSITY PRESS

New York

NEW YORK UNIVERSITY PRESS
New York
www.nyupress.org

References to Internet websites (URLs) were accurate at the time of writing. Neither the author nor New York University Press is responsible for URLs that may have expired or changed since the manuscript was prepared.

Library of Congress Cataloging-in-Publication Data
Names: Underman, Kelly, author.
Title: Feeling medicine : how the pelvic exam shapes medical training / Kelly Underman.
Description: New York : New York University Press, [2020] | Series: Biopolitics : medicine, technoscience, and health in the twenty-first century series | Includes bibliographical references and index.
Identifiers: LCCN 2019041471 | ISBN 9781479897780 (cloth) | ISBN 9781479893041 (paperback) | ISBN 9781479836338 (ebook) | ISBN 9781479878666 (ebook)
Subjects: LCSH: Gynecology—Study and teaching—United States. | Physicians—Training of—United States. | Pelvis—Examination—Social aspects—United States. | Human anatomy—Models—United States. | Gynecologist and patient—United States.
Classification: LCC RG143.A1 U84 2020 | DDC 618.071/173—dc23
LC record available at https://lccn.loc.gov/2019041471

New York University Press books are printed on acid-free paper, and their binding materials are chosen for strength and durability. We strive to use environmentally responsible suppliers and materials to the greatest extent possible in publishing our books.

Manufactured in the United States of America

10 9 8 7 6 5 4 3 2 1

Also available as an ebook

For Dad, who taught me to be curious.

CONTENTS

Introduction

The Quandary of the Sacred Vagina: Medical Education in a New Era

The anatomy lab has long held a fascinating and central position on the path to becoming a physician. And why not? Scholars of medical education and physicians have both written about how working with the cadaver prepares the medical student for this singular profession, in which personhood—for patient and trainee—is reworked or vacated entirely, death is a daily fact, and the body is cut into and opened up in ways that violate many deeply held cultural values. Commentators have noted that the anatomy lab also sets the model for the physician-patient relationship: a stoic expert applies knowledge to the inert and voiceless patient. Of course, none of these lessons is explicit. Trainees learn from their instructors and their peers about the so-called "soft skills" of being a physician from interactions with one another and everything that goes *un*said.

And yet, the anatomy lab is rapidly losing ground as the key mechanism for teaching trainees about the physician-patient relationship and the profession of medicine (Vinson 2019). Since the 1990s, the implicit and informal ways in which medical students were socialized have lost prominence in favor of explicit and formal systems of knowledge and practice that teach medical students how to become physicians. The rise of required courses on professionalism is just one such example, and one of the most visible. Attend any conference on health professions education today, and you will hear experts debate the most cutting-edge and scientifically vetted methods for producing the next generation of physicians.

With this shift toward the explicit, formal, and intensive has come a dramatic change in the profession's attitude toward feelings. In the old model of the anatomy lab, learning to suppress your horror, disgust, fear, or sadness was as central a lesson as learning the shapes and locations of organs. However, newer models of educating trainees take feelings head-on: medical students have memorial services to honor the humanity of their cadavers and grapple with their emotions around death and dying, attend art classes to develop their empathy, and, perhaps most tellingly, are judged on a portion of the United States Medical Licensing Exam (USMLE) on their ability to evoke and manage patient's feelings about their illnesses.

This shift is fascinating for a profession that has spent almost the entirety of the twentieth century cultivating detachment and dispassionate concern among its initiates. Nowhere is this shift more apparent than in teaching and learning the pelvic examination. In previous generations, medical students learned this exam on clinic patients who were given no opportunity to refuse. Medical students were taught to ignore their own and their patients' feelings about the exam, much in line with the model of expert-object established in the anatomy lab. In fact, patients who did have feelings about the exam—perhaps that the speculum hurt or that the exam reminded them of past trauma—were pathologized. Today's medical students now almost all learn the exam on the body of a trained and well-paid layperson who is simultaneously also their instructor. These laypeople emphasize not just the manual skills of inserting a speculum and checking the internal organs for disease, but also the interactional aspects of how to make patients feel safe, comfortable, and respected. In addition, they acknowledge the medical students' own feelings of anxiety or squeamishness and provide a supportive environment for trainees to make mistakes.

Learning about the body from a body that sits up and talks back is a markedly different kind of socialization than learning from the cadaver or the inert clinic patient. This new kind of pedagogy is embedded in a broader transformation in the profession to value feelings between and within physicians and patients. Conversations about empathy and burnout abound, even as metrics assessing the encounter, such as patient satisfaction scores, proliferate. No longer is the patient a passive object receiving the physician's expert knowledge. The patient is centered in the relationship, the patient is empowered, the patient is to be engaged in decision-making. There is clearly a new landscape about feelings in clinical medicine.[1]

This, finally, is how we make good doctors, isn't it? We have upended paternalism and replaced it with empowerment. We have leveled the power imbalance. We are making more resilient and compassionate physicians. Undoubtedly, paternalism is better left in the past, and treating patients like objects is detrimental to both patients' and physicians' wellbeing. But the power of medicine has not diminished. Indeed, health itself is increasingly a virtue that all patients are required to manage in order to maintain their wellbeing. More and more experts and forms of expertise guide our lives and tell us the kinds of people we should be and the ways that we should act with regard to our health. The patient, by sitting up and speaking back, is certainly empowered, but to what end? What are the consequences of this shift for how feelings are managed in clinical medicine? What kinds of people are we shaping medical trainees—and by extension, patients—to become? What are the norms and values embedded in this new professional landscape? And what are the points of resistance, the fissures and exclusions, the bodies that are left out?

In this book, I take up these questions by looking at the teaching and learning of the pelvic exam in gynecological teaching associate (GTA) programs. The pelvic exam is a fascinating case for understanding medical socialization today, as it involves a two-pronged navigation of feelings. It is about the emotions of physician and patient, but it is also about the embodied experience of sensation for both. The GTA program today has been shaped as well by the legacy of feminist health activism and the science-driven reform efforts of medical educators. While it is surely an exceptional experience—one or several one-to-three-hour workshops during all of medical school—it is embedded in and demonstrative of larger trends in medical education and, indeed, the medical profession.

I argue that teaching and learning the pelvic exam through the use of GTAs demonstrates the tension between the ever-presence of feelings and the drive toward standardization in twenty-first-century United States medical education. Learning the pelvic exam from a trained layperson prepares medical trainees to embody the changing values of the medical profession. As feelings have come to matter in new and complicated ways, medical educators and indeed the profession as a whole have developed scientific methods for measuring, modifying, and appropriating affect in the clinical setting. By *affect*, I mean the capacity of bodies to move, sense, and form connections with one another. These proliferating technologies serve to manage the behaviors of physicians and, by extension, patients. And yet, such affective capacities can never be fully captured by the tools of science. In short, I argue that teaching and learning the pelvic exam through the use of GTAs demonstrates how affect has instrumental value for upholding the cultural, political, and economic interests of the medical profession—and the forms of resistance possible therein.

"The Quandary of the Sacred Vagina": The Pelvic Exam and Medical Socialization

The pelvic exam is a cornerstone moment for many medical students. It is the first time they are required to touch a real human being in a sensitive and sexually charged area of the body in a professional manner. In a 2015 article in *Medical Education*, the premier journal for the titular discipline, a physician educator wondered about "the quandary of the sacred vagina": "Why does the female pelvic examination receive so much attention in medical education?" (Posner 2015:1179). Other examinations like the male abdominal "can be painful if performed improperly," yet the "female reproductive system occupies a special place in our curriculum." This physician educator argues that the combination of the vagina being a "private part" and the reproductive organs being internal to the body makes this examination unique among those that medical students must learn. As such, the pelvic exam can invoke a lot of anxiety for medical students. "The true benefit of the GTA experience may be in starting to overcome one's fear of harming someone" (Posner 2015:1180). These questions about hidden interiors of the body, sacred orifices, fear and harm, have long captured my attention as a sociologist.[2] What makes the vagina "sacred" enough to pose a quandary for medical students and educators? Given all the invasive and potentially painful techniques a medical student must learn to perform on another's body, how did it become possible that laypeople would voluntarily undergo this process—repeatedly? And why did medical educators agree that laypeople were the best method of instruction?

Prior to about the mid- to late 1980s, a medical student's first encounter with the pelvic exam would typically occur on an actual clinic patient, sometimes under anesthesia (Beckmann et al. 1985, 1992).[3] A majority—72 percent—of today's medical students in the United States will practice the exam on a GTA (Dugoff et al. 2016). While the focus of this book is on medical education in the United States, GTAs are also used commonly in Canada, Australia, and Scandinavian countries, and they are gaining popularity in Turkey, the United Kingdom, and elsewhere (Janjua et al. 2017; Sarmasoglu et al. 2016; Smith, Choudhury, and Clark 2015). GTA programs are one of a number of simulated patient experiences that medical students have; almost all physical exam skills are now taught on trained laypeople. Simulated patients are also used in the USMLE (also called the Step exams) that all medical students have to pass in order to practice medicine in the United States.[4] In this way, the growth of simulated patients—as in GTA programs—represents how medical education increasingly uses the tools of science to standardize how medical students learn to manage the physician-patient relationship.

For patients, the pelvic exam can very commonly be experienced at best as unpleasant and at worst as painful and frightening (Bloomfield et al. 2014). For almost seven decades it has been a once-yearly ritual for patients assigned female at birth.[5] Until the mid-2000s, it was used as a gatekeeping mechanism for allowing patients to access hormonal forms of contraception, thus linking patients' bodily autonomy with medical control of the body (Stewart et al. 2001). Notable exceptions to this include the Women's Health Movement of the 1960s and 1970s, which encouraged self- and group-based pelvic exams and performance art such as that of Annie Sprinkle (Kapsalis 1997).[6] But for most of us with vaginas, this exam invokes feelings of vulnerability, often magnified by the objectifying gaze of our physician.

At this point, you may be wondering, as a physician wondered in print in the *American Journal of Obstetrics and Gynecology*, "What kind of woman lets . . . novice medical students examine her?" (Kretzschmar 1978:373). Bound up in this question are all kinds of assumptions about sexuality, deviance, and masochism. Any person who has ever had a pelvic exam might immediately cross their legs and wonder why anyone would do this voluntarily and for money. Whenever I talk about my research, from professional conferences to cocktail parties, I am always greeted by surprise that this kind of thing even happens (let alone that I myself was once *that kind* of woman who let novice medical students examine me for money). When I speak to physicians about my work, almost every single one tells me with enthusiasm and respect about the GTA from whom they first learned the exam. *I was so nervous, and she made it so comfortable.*

This is exactly the reason why the pelvic exam—"the quandary of the sacred vagina"—receives so much attention in medical school. Indeed, after leaving medical school or residency, a physician may likely never perform this exam again. The routine pelvic exam is on the decline in the United States, now being performed every three to five years for most patients instead of every year. New technologies in the detection of cervical cancer–causing strains of the human papilloma virus (HPV) have made the cornerstone of the yearly pelvic exam, the Pap smear, less important if not soon to be obsolete. And yet, in 2016 alone, there were over 37 million office visits where a pelvic exam was performed (National Center for Health Statistics 2016). Its role in clinical practice extends beyond cancer detection, even if saving lives is its greatest success. The visual inspection and bimanual exam assess for sexually transmitted infections or endometriosis, and the speculum exam tests for vaginosis or allows for cervical biopsy. Thus, while your average physician is unlikely to practice the full exam as taught by GTAs on a regular basis, the GTA session itself remains a foundational moment in medical training.

GTA programs uniquely embody the tension between the drive toward science and standardization *and* the increasing centrality of care, relationality, and feeling in contemporary medical education. These programs arose as part of the wholesale shift toward standardized evaluation of clinical skills in the 1980s and 1990s, and yet they are fundamentally about feelings—about the experience of performing the exam and about what the exam feels like for patients to receive. GTAs teach from a checklist that was developed by experts on communication in the clinical encounter, even as their value resides in their highly detailed awareness of their own embodied sensations. In this way, the capacities of bodies to feel, sense, and relate, which I call *affect*, are caught in new and proliferating tensions as the medical profession transforms.

Medical Education and a Profession in Transition

GTA programs are the focus of this book, but they are indicative of larger trends in medical education and, indeed, in the profession in the United States. As I argue here, the medical profession has increasingly harnessed the affective capacities of its trainees and members in order to maintain its authority over patients. The reasons for this strategic deployment of affect has to do with profound structural transformations that occurred in healthcare and broader society in the United States during the 1970s and 1980s. To understand why these changes occurred and how medical education has grappled with them—especially in teaching and learning the pelvic exam—it is necessary to understand the social, political, and economic basis of the medical profession's authority.

Scientific knowledge is the bedrock of the medical profession's resilience in the face of structural and cultural changes in the landscape around it. This is due in large part to its ability to monopolize access to scientific knowledge about the body. Take, for example, its concerted efforts to shore up its authority in the nineteenth and early twentieth centuries, as its members began to regulate and standardize how trainees learned to become physicians.[7] Prior to these efforts, physicians were a loosely organized group whose training varied widely and whose effectiveness in treating illness even more so.[8] Two governing bodies—the American Medical Association (AMA), founded in 1847, and the Association of American Medical Colleges (AAMC), founded in 1876—issued requirements to its member schools regarding the training of students (Rothstein 1987). These tactics bolstered the authority of the profession and functioned to exclude those already marginalized in society.[9] This meant that women—especially women of color—who had for centuries taken care of pregnancy and childbirth, as well as many common ailments for their communities, were pushed out as the nascent medical profession sought to establish itself and claim the marketplace (McGregor 1998).

Advances in science and technology in the early twentieth century, such as the availability of sulfa (antibacterial) drugs and the discovery of blood types, further shored up the profession's authority. The growth of hospitals and increasing specialization among physicians led the AMA and other governing bodies to recommend more advanced training. As a result, the internship and residency became a crucial part of the elite physician's training. In addition, formal certification became commonplace. The AMA successfully lobbied all states to have licensing laws by 1900 and to require written exams for licensing by 1910 (Rothstein 1987). These included requiring four years' worth of courses and more rigorous education in the basic sciences.[10] The National Board of Medical Examiners (NBME) was founded in 1916 to supervise licensing examinations. The exam covered the basic and clinical sciences, as well as a practical component undertaken at the bedside. This brought previously unstandardized aspects of the physician-patient relationship, such as communication and decision-making, under the auspices of an increasingly scientific and institutional governing body.

During the middle of the twentieth century, the medical profession's drive toward science was fully entrenched as the strategy for maintaining professional dominance. The "art" of medicine became a science (Berg 1995). A solid proficiency in basic sciences was considered the most valuable for clinical reasoning and decision-making. Medical schools were increasingly tightly regulated by the AMA and the AAMC, so that admissions and curricular standards became more rigorous. In order to attract the best and brightest students, these schools readily complied with such standards. Uniformity of licensing procedures and examinations across the country was intended to ensure that only those deemed totally proficient could practice medicine. Moreover, medical training was extended beyond the four years of medical school into internships and residencies. Specialization became the routine rather than the exception, and advances in science and technology continually challenged medical schools and physicians to adapt.

During the 1960s and 1970s, a number of structural transformations shifted the relationship between the medical profession and the public that it purported to serve. The emergence of managed care and patient consumerism reorganized the economic structure of medicine. The advent of health maintenance organizations under federal law in 1973 introduced benefits and drawbacks that radically altered the provision of healthcare in the United States. Managed care involves negotiations between insurance companies and providers to control costs, such as limiting the length of hospital stays and denying unnecessary tests or procedures. As a result, hospital stays declined rapidly during the 1970s, as did the length of the routine clinical encounter. With the evolution of managed care into such health insurance plans as preferred provider organizations, healthcare became a product that the savvy consumer should shop for through choices of providers, hospitals, and clinics. Patients started to think and act more like consumers than docile subjects. In addition, patients became more active in other ways. The patient health movements that emerged in the 1970s and proliferate today can be seen as both a kind of consumeristic activism and a push-back on the professional authority of physicians during a time of generalized declining trust in experts.[11] The Women's Health Movement, which helped reshape teaching and learning the pelvic exam during the 1970s and 1980s, is one such example.

As the type of patient changed during the 1970s, the type of medical student also changed. Women began entering medical schools during the 1970s and early 1980s in high numbers. Prior to 1970, women made up less than a tenth of medical students. By 1975, women accounted for one-fifth of medical students and one-third by 1985 (AAMC 2016). By the early 1990s, women made up roughly half of all medical students, and this continues to be the case. Similarly, relatively more people of color entered medical school in the 1970s and 1980s, primarily those of Asian descent, although since the 1990s and 2000s, Latinx and Black students have been making up larger portions of the medical student body (Lee and Franks 2010). These transformations shook up the culture of medical schools, as educators had to grapple with the gendered and racialized constructions of who got to count as a legitimate scientific expert.

With these structural transformations came an intensified interest in the medical profession's Holy Grail for controlling access to scientific knowledge: the licensing exam. Throughout the 1970s, licensing requirements for physicians became increasingly more stringent.[12] Oral exams for hospital house-staff (residents) were eliminated in 1970 and replaced with a written test. The largest change occurred in 1992 with the requirement of the United States Medical Licensing Exam (USMLE) through a collaboration between the National Board of Medical Examiners (NBME) and the Federation of State Medical Boards (FSMB).[13] As I demonstrate in this book, this introduced a new expert apparatus that governed what was considered appropriate professional behavior between physicians and patients, especially with regard to emotion. This also meant that one-off experiences such as the pelvic exam became important opportunities for medical students to practice communication and interpersonal skills that they needed in order to pass high-stakes testing.

Out of the patient activism of the 1970s and the reorganization of how healthcare is paid for emerged a reconceptualization of the debate about the physician-patient relationship and the role of feelings in medicine. During most of the twentieth century, the prevailing form of emotion in medicine was one of detached concern or affective neutrality. Renee Fox's (1979) path-breaking work demonstrated how medical trainees strove to maintain emotional distance in the face of suffering and death. This was to ensure the centrality of science: while physicians were expected to be sympathetic toward patients, any further kind of emotional engagement was thought to cloud judgment and introduce bias into the clinical encounter. As recently as the late 1980s, detached concern has been explicitly socialized into medical students through formal and informal means, especially during crucial experiences such as the pelvic exam (Smith and Kleinman 1989).

However, during the 1990s, new constellations of knowledge reordered the relationship between science and affect as medical educators reconsidered the role of feelings in the clinical encounter (Underman and Hirshfield 2016). For example, clinical empathy is a model in which physicians are urged to consider patients' emotions—and their own emotions—when making medical decisions (Halpern 2011). Rather than viewing emotion as a source of bias to be reasoned away and avoided, clinical empathy makes the emotional connection a physician might feel with a patient part of clinical practice. In this way, feeling *for* and *with* patients, rather than the cultivation of detachment and emotional distance, becomes a core component of a good physician. This shift toward attending to one's own feelings and the feelings of patients is nowhere more evident than in teaching and learning the pelvic exam, which forms the cornerstone of my argument in this book—namely, that how GTAs teach medical students to engage with patients' feelings reflects a largescale shift in how medical authority is exercised on and through the affective capacities of patients and physicians.

The "professionalism movement" in medical education also began in the late 1990s and has accelerated so that professionalism is now a "third-pillar" in most medical school curricula (with the sciences and clinical skills being the first two).[14] Classes, workshops, and other formal parts of the curricula make aspects of professionalism such as medical ethics, the physician-patient relationship, and clinical reasoning explicit requirements of medical school. Professionalism is sometimes framed as the outward expressions of respect, compassion, and so forth, for patients and colleagues. It is often fostered through exercises that involve reflexivity, such as reading poetry, free-writing or journaling, taking photos or painting, or speaking with a mentor. In this way, learning the pelvic exam with a GTA is exemplary of these new technologies for cultivating professionalism and its attendant affective capacities.

Thus, by the dawn of the twenty-first century, the tension between science and affect was being articulated in new ways and with new consequences in medical education. Professionalism has become an explicit concern among medical educators. Medical students experience more overt and intentional efforts than ever before to socialize them into the profession. Not only are medical students taught clinical skills and trained to embody new sets of values, but they are tested on them as well. These shifting standards respond as much to changing expectations from the public as to corporate hospital models that track metrics such as patient satisfaction and physician efficiency.[15] This book traces the ways new subjectivities for both physicians and patients are increasingly being produced through modification of the body's capacities to feel, sense, and relate. My conceptual framework draws together literature on expertise in biopolitical regimes—including how expertise "makes up" subjects of governance—with literature on affective economies. Taken together, these sets of literature show how expert knowledge and practice balance the social and cultural forces that emphasize care and compassion in clinical medicine with economic and political forces that demand the continued power and authority of the medical profession. These transformations are nowhere as evident in medical education as in the ways in which teaching and learning the pelvic exam has been reorganized.

Contemporary Clinical Governmentality

Since the 1970s, we have witnessed rapid and far-reaching transformations in the medical profession. The rise of informed consent and patient consumerism have meant that the physician-patient relationship has changed to emphasize a more flattened out rather than hierarchical exchange (Clarke et al. 2003; Reeder 1972). Technological advances, evidence-based medicine, and the electronic health record have reorganized medical knowledge (Clarke et al. 2003; Ebeling 2016; Joyce 2008; Reich 2012; Timmermans and Angell 2001; Timmermans and Oh 2010). Institutional pressures such as managed care, corporatization of healthcare, and the growth of the pharmaceutical industry and direct-to-consumer marketing have curtailed the autonomy of physicians (Bell and Figert 2012; Clarke et al. 2003). These transformations can all broadly be situated within the conceptual framework of biomedicalization, which sociologist Adele Clarke and her colleagues (2003) developed to account for the bottom-up and inside-out reorganization of medical knowledge and practice due to the proliferation of science and technology. And yet, despite these transformations, sociologists have only recently begun reconsidering the nature of professional dominance in healthcare (Vinson 2016). In this book, I use a case involving the teaching and learning the pelvic exam in medical education to understand the larger values and norms of the profession of medicine as it responds to these structural and institutional forces. Following theorists of biomedicalization, I situate the nature of contemporary medical authority within a neo-Foucauldian framework that conceptualizes power as productive and multifaceted. A neo-Foucauldian analysis also links the medical profession and how it shapes the behavior and personhood of its participants (physician and patient) to broader state and economic forces that structure our lives.

From the work of philosopher and historian Michel Foucault I draw on the concept of biopolitics to analyze the dual relationship between the production of knowledge about populations and the management of individual bodies as a form of social control (Foucault 1994, 1995). As Foucault famously wrote, biopolitics is a form of political rationality in which the state fosters or enables life *or* disallows it to the point of death (Foucault 1990). Family-planning programs in the early twentieth century are a classic example that Foucault himself used. The state gathered scientific data on the population in order to encourage the "right" forms of reproduction among middle-class white heterosexual married couples, while pursuing eugenics programs for those deemed "unfit" to reproduce: people of color, the poor, the disabled, et cetera. In this way, the knowledge/power nexus targets the body and its productive capacities in order to shape society as a whole. Indeed, what makes biopolitics a useful concept is that it reframes power as not only or not just prohibitive. Power does not suppress through applications of force in biopolitics; instead, it is productive. Systems of knowledge shape individuals' behaviors, attitudes, hopes, and aspirations. Thus, scholars began writing about the power of the medical profession as it pertains to this form of biopolitical governmentality (Armstrong 1983, 1995; Turner 1995, 1997), by which I mean this form of shaping populations through the acquisition and deployment of knowledge.

In a biopolitical analysis, power is conceived not so much as being centered in institutional spaces and wielded by individuals but as a productive force that operates through forms of knowledge. One outcome of this shift toward a Foucauldian or biopolitical understanding of the medical profession is that instead of speaking of experts, we can now speak of expertise. The former is concerned with the socially valued properties of the individual, which make that person an expert, whereas the latter considers the practices, knowledges, and tools that mark as distinct a body of expertise (Eyal 2013). As social theorist Nikolas Rose argues variously in his work on expertise in late modern capitalism, the exercise of governance is no longer necessarily organized through society or the state, but through an increasing array of forms of expertise. Through the truth claims of expertise, people can be governed "at arms' length": "Political rule would not itself set out the norms of individual conduct, but would install and empower a variety of 'professionals' who would, investing them with authority to act as experts in the devices of social rule" (Rose 1993:285). A very basic and low-stakes example of this that I use with undergraduates is about dental hygiene: we do not brush our teeth every day because it is a law; we do so because a professional (a dentist) equipped with a special body of knowledge (dental medicine) teaches us that this is the best way to live our lives (remaining cavity-free). Likewise, the number of such professionals who shape and guide our behavior in relationship to health and illness is proliferating. Physicians now work alongside advanced practice nurses, physician's assistants, health coaches, clinical psychologists and social workers, and so on and so forth, in order to manage disease, as well as to promote health itself to the population as a moral obligation. These health experts all operate within the *episteme* of medicine, meaning that the physician is not *the* only pathway to scientific knowledge about disease, illness, and health; rather, a network of practices, knowledges, and tools functions in the service of biopolitical governance.

A key aspect of this shift is that experts no longer exercise direct control via discipline. Instead, individuals are increasingly targeted by the productive operations of power to become self-responsible and self-governing (Metzl and Kirkland 2010; Rose 2009). In these new forms of governance through expertise, we are not only obligated to get professional help when we become sick, but also encouraged to constantly and actively monitor ourselves to maintain our health. To return to my example of dental hygiene, notices from the dental office to show up for our six-month cleaning and the institutional site of the dentist's office (the waiting room, the chair, the lights and tools) serve to *discipline* us to accept the dentist's role as an arbiter of dental expertise. But it is the equipping us with knowledge about dental hygiene via public health campaigns about brushing and flossing that turns us into good dental citizens. *Not* brushing thus takes on a moral quality: tell someone you decided not to brush your teeth this morning and see how what the response is. Congratulations, you have taken medical authority into your own body. This process works for all areas of health and illness. Diet, exercise, taking medications for our anxiety and vitamins to strengthen our bones, all function to promote health as a moral obligation. This is what I mean by biopolitical governance making us self-responsible.

However, this shift should not be taken as evidence that, because the medical profession no longer has a stranglehold on scientific knowledge, we as patients are liberated, but rather that control operates variously through knowledge. No longer being beholden to institutional spaces of power and direct exercises of authority does not mean we are free to live as we want. Instead, it means that expertise serves to continuously modify and guide the choices we make about our lives. Thus, a study of expertise "opens up for investigation the complexity and diversity of the relations between authorities and subjects, and the ways in which such practices have not suppressed freedom but, on the contrary, sought to 'make up' subjects capable of exercising a regulated freedom and caring for themselves as free subjects" (Rose 1993:288). The burden of biopolitical power is now placed onto individuals through processes of turning them into the kinds of people who can and will act as "good" subjects. It is this process of crafting subjects through the sharing and spread of biomedical knowledge that I am concerned with in this book. I explore how both physicians and patients are "made up" by experts and the spread of expert knowledge through the GTA session in order to explicate the norms and values of "good" members of our society.

And yet, the major social institutions around which Foucault framed his theory are breaking down (Deleuze 1992). The clinic no longer operates as the only way in which the norms and values of medicine become embodied in patients. Indeed, the shift from discipline to control that has more broadly reshaped the institutions and structures of contemporary society has also reshaped medical authority. In societies of control, power circulates ubiquitously and relies on modification and modulation rather than discipline (Deleuze 1992). In this way, theories of control, rather than discipline, better account for the circulation of "health itself" in society and the new ways in which patients increasingly are self-responsible and self-monitoring, instead of simply or only submitting themselves to the authority of the physician in ways enabled by the physical environment of the clinic. Although work on biopolitics has captured the transformation in the nature of biomedical power, it has not fully accounted for the mechanisms by which patients and physicians are transformed as subjects. This is where my concept of this book intervenes: expert systems of knowledge and practice produce contemporary subjects of biopolitics by acting on and through affect.

The Affective Turn and Clinical Medicine

We are in the midst of an "affective turn" in the social sciences, cultural studies, and the humanities, in which new attention is being paid to embodied forms of feeling.[16] Affect is the capacities of bodies to feel, sense, and relate. I draw from a Deleuzian tradition, in which affect can be thought of an intensity lived at the level of the body.[17] Given that teaching and learning the pelvic exam in the GTA session involves circulations of sensation within the body and between bodies, and given how charged this exam is by feelings of shame, anxiety, and disgust, this concept is essential to my analysis. Conceptualizing affect in this way captures embodiment and our capacities to form connections with the social and material world around us, as well as the new ways in which power works on and through our bodies under scientific and capitalist regimes.

Why would I use the term "affect" instead of "emotion," since there is such a rich literature on emotion in sociology already? For example, Arlie Hochschild's (2012) canonical book, *The Managed Heart*, introduced the concept of emotional labor, which is work that requires the management of one's own emotions (feeling rules) and emotional expressions (display rules) in order to induce or suppress emotions in others, usually paying clients. This concept has been influential in many fields and has made its way into the medical education literature. However, a growing body of literature is starting to recast emotional labor in the terms of affective labor to better capture the nature of work in late modern capitalism (Hardt 1999; Weeks 2007). For example, what is being produced by the programmers who write the algorithms that guide what stories show first in your Facebook feed? This is not quite emotional labor. Instead, it is about producing emotional or affective states in order to produce capital—that is, money for advertisers.

While affect and emotion are interrelated concepts, they have important differences and I use them differently throughout the book. Put simply, affect is the pre-social, pre-linguistic, pre-conscious *experience*, while emotion is the individualized, named, recognized *state* (Gould, 2009). Brian Massumi writes, "An emotion is . . . the sociolinguistic fixing of the quality of an experience which is from that point onward defined as personal" (2002:28). Or: "An emotion or feeling is a recognized affect" (Massumi 2002:61). This may seem like splitting theoretical hairs, but this difference is important for the other properties of affect that make it a useful concept. Unlike emotion, affect is not fixed or contained inside one body of one individual. Instead, it circulates between bodies, between signs, between material objects and discourses. Because of this inability to fully capture and contain affect, affect has the property of a verb: it *does* things. It moves, it connects, it severs. This property of affect is what I find most useful for understanding the embodied nature of medicine. Affect allows for physicians and patients to "move with and be moved by" (Myers 2012) one another and the spaces, objects, and tools of the clinic. In my analysis, I follow sociologist Deborah Gould

(2009) in using the word *affect* to describe this vital force and the word *emotion* to describe the recognized state.

Affect is produced and circulated in social relationships. In her masterful work on the social production of emotion, Sara Ahmed contends that affect is produced in historically specific circulations among subjects, which she calls *affective economies*. "In such affective economies, emotions do things, and they align individuals with communities" (Ahmed 2004:119). For example, hate for a feared outsider binds a nation together as one. The collective grief or rage experienced by a marginalized community moves its members to action in pursuit of social justice (Gould 2009). In this way, affect circulates through sideways or "sticky" associations and generates the surfaces and boundaries of individual and collective bodies. Due to the weight of history, some bodies are "stickier" than others and accumulate more affective charge. Thus, capacities to experience and display emotion, and the resultant modes of embodiment, are produced in specific historical and cultural contexts and become bound up with the political and economic structures in which they are valued. In this way, we can more fully parse the different ways in which communities of color, for example, experience the physician-patient relationship compared with white people.[18] Or we can better account for why Black men self-report the highest rates of empathy of any group in standardized tests of physician-patient communication and yet are rated the lowest, while white women consistently perform the best (Berg et al. 2015). Some bodies simply come into medical school with different affective charges due to historical and material conditions of social life. Stereotypes about white women as nice and kind or Black men as dangerous and aggressive become layered into the body as affects that circulate in these spaces.

Because of its capacity to "surface" bodies and create boundaries, affect is increasingly becoming the target of regimes of governmentality. By this I mean that affect is becoming both the target of and the tool through which the conduct of the population is guided, controlled, and disciplined.[19] The emerging literature on affect and control demonstrates the role of affect in contemporary processes of biopolitics (Anderson 2012; Clough 2003, 2008; Clough et al. 2007). Accordingly, biopolitical power acts on and through affect, making affect both the target of power and its condition for existence. Power acts on and through us by modifying and managing our lived intensities of the social world and thus our emotion. Modifications of how people feel assist in the production of certain kinds of subjects: how we are made to feel shapes the kinds of people we want—and are able—to be. In biomedicine, hope or trust makes patients into willing consumers (Brown 2015). A whole range of psychological research on "person perception ability" links the ability of physicians to successfully judge a patient's emotional state with patient satisfaction and compliance.[20] This also means that affect has an economic value, either directly or indirectly. Directly, we see affect as a commodity in self-help and motivational industries, where the imperative is to live happily. Indirectly, we see it in the rise of "do what you love" directives—wherein "doing what you love" is more important than economic stability—and of "self-care" economies at work. For example, in the health professions, "self-care" in the form of exercise, journaling, bubble baths, and so forth, is promoted in place of addressing structural issues that lead to burnout. Affect is thus endlessly exploited in the service of capitalism.[21] In this way, affective governance is a new mode of producing physicians and patients under corporatized regimes of for-profit healthcare.

Affective Governance in Medical Education

By linking theories of affect with those of governmentality, I argue that not just emotion but our capacities to sense, relate, and feel are bound up in the workings of power via deployments of expertise.[22] In this way, I contend with a conceptualization of *affective governance in medical education*.[23] I use this phrase to capture all of the ways in which affect has become a target of contemporary forces of governance in the training of the next generation of medical students, as well as the forms of resistance available within such strategies. Further, my analysis considers affective governance in medical education across several scales of action.

First, I am interested in the *regimes* of affect that characterize medical education. I draw on a Foucauldian notion of regimes (Bell 2009; Foucault 1982, 1995; Klawiter 2008; Moseby 2017), which considers the historically specific and temporally bounded processes by which systems of knowledge and discourse are formed. Regimes are the particular kinds of mechanisms that exist in a given time and place and govern what is true or not based on that locality's means of knowing. We can see these at work in how affect is known in specific ways in medical education and increasingly incorporated in its professional projects. I opened this introduction with some examples of the ways that medical students' feelings matter in new ways. We can see a new regime of affect at work in concern about burnout, in mindfulness and meditation training in medical schools, in standardized licensing questions that evaluate medical students' abilities to manage their feelings and their patients' feelings. Even debates about the anatomy lab demonstrate this new regime of affect: costly and environmentally questionable as cadavers are, they're still important for medical students to acquire the feel of working with human tissues (Prentice 2013). A concept related to regimes of affect is *economies of affect* in medical education. Economies of affect are those zones or spaces within which affects circulate and are valued by expert knowledge (Ahmed 2004; Richard and Rudnyckyj 2009). Economies are essentially systems of management that value affective capacities within the structural or institutional spaces that they circulate in or flow through. While regimes are macro-level, I see economies as being more meso-level. Put another way, while regimes capture the changes in knowledge and organization in medical education around affect, economies capture the interpersonal or site-specific dynamics of affective flows.

Second, I am interested in the ways in which subjects of these new regimes of affective governance in medical education take up these regimes into their own bodies. I use the concept of *technologies of affect* to capture this. I define technologies of affect as those knowledges, practices, techniques, and discourses that seek to measure, manage, harness, and produce the affective capacities of medical students, and by extension patients. Technologies are those systems of knowledges and kinds of practices that enable larger structures of power to shape the conduct or behaviors of individual subjects. For example, in *Discipline and Punish*, Foucault traces the emergence of the prison as a kind of technology, comprised of physical environment, timetables for prisoner activity, ideas and knowledges about "rehabilitation," behavior and attitude of guards, and so forth, which shaped the prisoner into a certain—reformed—kind of person. One way to think of technologies is as instruments (in the forms of knowledges, discourses, and practices) that link macro-level strategies of governance with individuals. Foucault wrote of discipline as a key mechanism of power by which the major intuitions in society (such as the prison, the clinic, or the school) shape the behavior of its members.

In biomedicine, the practices, knowledges, and discourses that make up technologies of affect modify and mobilize the embodied capacities to feel of both physicians and patients. Physicians are targeted by these technologies in order to become more efficient workers while also maintaining authority in the encounter. Patients are targeted in order to produce the kinds of people who will take up biomedical expertise into their own bodies to manage their own health and wellness and participate in economies as workers and consumers. The concept of technologies of affect accounts for transformations in the profession of medicine in which physicians increasingly rely on using emotion to ensure patient trust and compliance. In this way, it updates theories of professional dominance for the new landscape of health logics under capitalism formed by biomedicalization. Technologies of affect account for the mutuality of subject formation in biomedicine, so that sociological work on both professional socialization and on the disciplining of patients are linked.

I will describe a number of technologies of affect in medical education, but my particular focus is on the role of simulation, using the case of teaching and learning the pelvic exam. Simulation, as in the GTA session, is produced within the expertise of medical education, and it guides and shapes the behaviors and attitudes of medical students. However, the techniques and skills that medical students are taught through simulated encounters such as the GTA session shape not only their subjectivities as future physicians. Medical students learn sets of practices that are intended to also shape the behaviors and attitudes of patients. The key target of intervention in these interlinked sets of practices is affect. By shaping the bodily capacities of medical students—and by extension, patients—the expertise of medical education seeks to produce subjects of these new forms of biomedical power. Thus, technologies of affect seek to (re)establish the authority of the medical profession by shaping patients' emotional selves.

Outline of the Book

The data for this book come from a qualitative study of GTA programs at three medical schools in Chicago. Between 2011 and 2013, I conducted interviews with three groups of stakeholders: GTAs and their program coordinators, medical faculty, and medical students. I also collected educational data from 2011 to 2019. These sources included medical journal articles, syllabi and lecture notes, meeting minutes and center reports, materials used to train GTAs and those handed out to students, and so forth; in total, I had over a thousand pages to sort through. From 2015 to 2017, I was a postdoctoral research associate in a department of medical education, which exposed me to the larger practical and research apparatus of the discipline. Finally, and perhaps most crucially, I worked as a GTA in two major cities between the years of 2005 and 2015. I would not have known that such a job exists without having done it—most people who have not gone to medical school do not. In addition, my questions about expertise, the politics of care, and the body are intimately shaped and inspired by the decade I spent doing this work. I address these issues in the methodological appendix.

In chapter 1, I provide a brief history of how sensitive exams have been taught and the debates within and beyond medical schools about how to teach these. I then consider the role of the Women's Health Movement and the rise of medical education research in the formation of the GTA program. I argue that feminist practices of care have transformed how the pelvic exam is taught in medical education, even as medical education researchers coopted these practices to serve the interests of the medical profession. Thus, in demonstrating the rise of affective governance in medical education, I also consider the instrumental ends that affects like caring and empathy serve. I continue this theme in chapter 2, where I contextualize the growth of GTA programs within a larger trend in medical education toward standardizing clinical skills education. I argue that medical education research produces technologies of affect in order to shape the conduct of physicians and patients. I use simulated patients and the communication and interpersonal skills checklist that GTAs use to evaluate medical students' performance as examples of such technologies.

In chapter 3, I argue that GTAs perform a kind of intimate labor that relies upon care and attentiveness to their bodies, their coworkers' bodies, and the bodies and emotions of their students. I analyze the accounts that GTAs give for their motivations to do this work and some of the challenges they face on the job. In doing so, I demonstrate how GTAs' intimate labor is intended to produce caring ties between future physicians and their patients, and thus to produce certain kinds of expert subjects who can uphold medical authority in the era of corporatized healthcare. I continue this theme in chapter 4, where I argue that the seemingly artificial context of the GTA session prepares medical students to embody the norms and values of a changing profession. I analyze medical students' accounts of the pelvic exam as a pivotal moment in their training and link these to how medical educators describe the importance of this foundational encounter.

In chapter 5, I turn my attention to how GTAs train medical students to become aware of novel sensations in their own bodies in order to locate and make an object of attention out of the internal reproductive anatomy. I argue that this attention to "feeling with" the body posits feeling as a collectivized, embodied practice, in which affects circulate within and between bodies, and I explore the implications of this concept and practice for theories of clinical perception. Finally, in chapter 6, I explore another subject-making practice by analyzing how GTAs teach medical students techniques of patient empowerment in the pelvic exam. I argue that patient empowerment represents another technology of affect, this one intended to produce patients as "partners," subjects who are responsible for participating, and obligated to participate, in the maintenance of their own health. I consider how these technologies construct the ideal patient—and who is left out by them.

In the conclusion, I revisit my argument about affective governance in medical education. I consider some of the implications of theorizing affective governance for healthcare. I demonstrate forms of resistance to normalizing technologies of affect and argue for reforms in medical education that can challenge the ways in which affect becomes instrumentalized under for-profit corporate healthcare regimes.

Thus, taken together, this book uses the case of teaching and learning the pelvic exam in contemporary United States medical education to understand the complicated ways in which affect—that is, bodily capacities to sense, relate, and form connections—are appropriated by expert knowledges and practices in the service of maintaining professional dominance and biopolitical control. The coalescing of this new regime is evident in how feminist practices have challenged sexist and racist practices in teaching and learning the pelvic exam, even as these same practices have been coopted by medical education. In this way, in chapter 1 and throughout the book, I hold the positive impacts of feminist politics of care alongside their exclusions and limitations, demonstrating how medicine simultaneously is transformed by and coopts interventions and challenges.

1

The Pelvic Exam and the Politics of Care

[A faculty member] would go down to the public clinic, manually select a woman, say, "You're going to come upstairs and teach the pelvic exam." Not "are you?" or "will you?" "You are." He would completely cover the patient with drapes, including the head. [He would] go into the exam room and the students were probing down this anonymous vagina and roll her out. Then he'd give her money.
—Charles, MD, medical faculty

I like the fact that they're [GTAs] sitting up, that they're able to see what the practitioner's doing and not laying back where they can't see anything. . . . They feel by training young people early on and getting them in the habit of proper communication and touch . . . [and] different techniques that . . . help to make the whole experience . . . less scary . . . [like] you're going to look forward to going to your provider.
—Heather, program coordinator

These two quotations represent two different regimes of practice for teaching and learning the pelvic exam in medical school, one before and one after the introduction of gynecological teaching associates.[1] In the first, Charles, a senior physician, reflects on how the previous generation of medical students at his university were taught the pelvic exam. A woman waiting in a public clinic for perhaps something completely unrelated would be forced to have medical students examine her in exchange for her "free" healthcare. Her subjectivity was removed as her body became reduced to an "anonymous vagina" that medical students would "prob[e] down" in the presence of their instructor; this woman would literally become an object under the medical gaze.[2] In the second quotation,

Heather, the coordinator of a GTA program, reflects on how medical students are taught the pelvic exam today. Instead of an "anonymous vagina" coerced into the exam, well-paid volunteers now use their bodily expertise to train medical students on more than just the most basic components of the exam. These women, in contrast to those in Charles's example, sit up and look their trainees face to face. They teach about communication skills such as offering a verbal warning before you make intimate contact with a patient's genitals. Emotion is never mentioned in Charles's example, though it does show how affects of disrespect toward and dehumanization of patients are cultivated in medical trainees. In Heather's, the patient's emotion is centered in the process of cultivating affects of attentiveness and empathy in trainees: the exam should be "less scary," even to the point of it being something patients look forward to having. There is a distinct ethos of care in Heather's description that is lacking in Charles's.

I argue in this chapter that teaching and learning the pelvic exam in United States medical education has been transformed by feminist practices of care, even as these same practices have been coopted in order to serve the interests of physicians and medical educators. In making this argument, I also demonstrate how the disruptive potential of affect is managed by new strategies of governance in medical education. The background for this chapter is the incidental convergence of several histories: during the 1970s and 1980s, the Women's Health Movement, medical education research, and transformations in biomedicine altered one another's trajectories and changed how the pelvic exam is taught to medical students and, thus, the pelvic exam itself. I use the development of the program at one university as a case study to show how these dynamics played out on the ground, at the same time that large structural forces were operating at the national (and to a lesser extent the international) scale to challenge existing practices. As I follow these historical shifts, I trace what changed and what stayed the same in teaching and learning the pelvic exam. I claim that the way that these three histories converge on the pelvic exam demonstrates the transformations that are possible to the material practices of medical education through feminist activism—and those that remain untenable given structures of knowledge and power in biomedicine.

In particular, I follow transformations with regard to practices of care in clinical medicine. The two quotations with which I opened the chapter demonstrate two very different forms of relating to patients in teaching and learning the pelvic exam. The physician in Charles's example probably did care about patients at his clinic inasmuch as he felt it was his mission to treat and prevent disease. But he certainly did not demonstrate the kind of care for patients that Heather's GTAs do in their commitment to making the pelvic exam if not something "to look forward to," at least "less scary." Here, I use the concept of assemblage to analyze how the politics of care have been articulated in the pelvic exam across its history. What makes the concept of the assemblage useful is that it describes both the "hanging together" of diverse, multilayered elements, as well as the opposite: the continual "lines of flight" or pulling apart of these elements.[3] I consider the pelvic exam as an assemblage in order to account for biomedical discourse, the materiality of bodies and tools, the social relations within the encounter, and so forth, all coexisting within this fraught practice. Throughout this chapter I draw attention to what components of the assemblage are being reworked in any given situation in order to trace how care has been worked into the pelvic exam.

I am informed by the feminist work in science and technology studies on care as an affectively charged "attachment or commitment to something" (de la Bellacasa 2011:89–90). In these literatures, care invokes notions of material doing, by which I mean that caring involves direct engagement with the material world, with its tools and practices, as it pertains to something that a person or group cares about.[4] Thus, throughout this chapter, think of care when I discuss it as an affective engagement in practice. To care about someone or something is to invest some part of oneself emotionally, to be attentive to and engaged with the object of one's care. In this way, care has had to be assembled into the pelvic exam through feminist actions. And yet, due to the standardizing and objectively oriented goals of medical education and, more broadly, biomedicine itself, feminist means of caring can always only be partially assembled into the pelvic exam. I identify simulation as the key technology through which feminist practices of care are incorporated into medical education and show how caring practices bump up against structural forces that dictate who, what, and how care can be enfolded into biomedicine.

Moreover, to care is to make choices about what else one is *not* caring about. Care "is a selective mode of attention" (Martin, Myers, and Viseu

2015:627) in that by making space for some issues, people, or things, it excludes others. This raises the issue of a *politics* of care. "Practices of care are always shot through with asymmetrical power relations: who has the power to care? Who has the power to define what counts as care and how it should be administered?" (Martin, Myers, and Viseu 2015:627). In this way, care cannot be thought of as always innocent, always positive, always beneficial for all. Rather, care "organizes, classifies, and disciplines bodies[;] . . . care makes palpable how justice for some can easily become injustice for others" (Martin, Myers, and Viseu 2015:627). The politics of care are "entangled in the complex devaluing and valuing of care, even as care is repeatedly promised as a source of potential emancipation and alternative technoscience" (Murphy 2015:724). Thus, when analyzing practices of cares, scholars must be attentive to (should I say *care*ful of?) easy promises of liberation through the incorporation of care and must instead constantly be aware of the exclusions and other arrangements that make some lives less livable. As I show in this chapter, the politics of care in teaching and learning the pelvic exam are entangled in the complicated histories of exclusion between biomedicine and gender, sexuality, and race. This links to my larger argument in this book about the ways in which affective capacities (of which care is one) are harnessed and manipulated by governance strategies in medical education: caring about patients in the way that is being taught reinforces medical authority across an uneven terrain of power in an era of corporatized healthcare.

The Biopolitics of the Pelvic Exam

The pelvic exam is a collection of gestures, actions, tools, words, and bodies of knowledge—both scientific and experiential. Each one of these components is imbued with history—not only the physician or patient's own experience, but the social and historical contexts that shaped it as it came into being. What arose as a routine technology for the biomedical disciplining of gendered and racialized bodies has become a collaborative practice shaped by contemporary discourses about the physician-patient relationship. Care has been incorporated into or absent from it in complex and contradictory ways. Understanding where the pelvic exam comes from is crucial to understanding the forms of protest surrounding it and its continual modulation through the interventions of medical educators and patient health movements. The pelvic exam's troubling history is rooted in racist and (hetero)sexist exploitation of bodies. While midwives have long examined pregnant people's bodies and sex workers have historically been subjected to physical inspection in the name of hygiene, the pelvic exam as a biomedical practice involving visual, manual, and speculum examination arose in the mid-nineteenth century with the nascent medical specialty of gynecology (McGregor 1998). Gynecology emerged out of obstetrics, as physicians increasingly identified diseases of the reproductive system or injuries due to difficult labor and delivery. Its foundational tool, the speculum, exemplifies its problematic origins (Barker-Benfield 2004; Snorton 2017; Washington 2006). French midwife Marie Boivin and French physician Joseph Claude Anselme Récamier are both credited with developing the bivalve speculum at about the same time, in 1825 (Ricci 1949). However, the speculum spread in the European medical communities in part because of public viewings at hospitals involving sex workers. Curious members of the medical community would watch as sex workers were forced to undergo public speculum examinations (Lee 1851; Ricci 1949).[5]

In the United States, the "father" of modern gynecology, J. Marion Sims, invented the forerunner of the "duckbill" speculum used today by exploiting the bodies of enslaved Black women (Owens 2017; Snorton 2017; Washington 2006). Sims was a pioneer in gynecological surgery, particularly of fistulas, which are vaginal openings or tears that allow urine or fecal matter to leak into the vagina. They were—and still are—debilitating conditions that need treatment, yet the methods Sims used demonstrate medicine's history of racist exploitation in the name of progress. Sims performed experimental surgeries on enslaved women without using anesthesia, even after anesthesia became routine. This was because Sims, like many, believed that Black people do not experience pain the way that white people do as a result of the brutalizing conditions of their enslavement (Owens 2017).[6] From these experiments on Lucy, Anarcha, Betsey, and almost thirty other enslaved Black women,[7] Sims developed the forerunner of today's speculum out of two spoons used to hold the open the vagina. The speculum thus allowed physicians better access to the interior organs of the body and became a material tool for expanding biopolitical control over certain kinds of bodies.

During the twentieth century, the pelvic exam became more commonplace as the relationship between medical authority and gendered (and racialized) bodies changed. The routine pelvic exam rose to prominence in the early part of the century with the invention of the Pap smear and its promotion through public health agencies (Casper and Clarke 1998; Löwy 2010). This tool served to expand the reach of biopolitics by coding reproductive bodies as always already at risk and in need of medical surveillance. During this time, the pelvic exam shifted from being about locating disease toward the maintenance of health via regular screening. With this shift, this form of discipline became about more than health—it also became about reinforcing (hetero)sexist discourses about reproductive bodies.[8]

During the middle part of the century—the so-called Golden Age of Doctoring—the premarital pelvic exam was made compulsory both by social norms and, in most states, by law.[9] During this exam, which was ostensibly about reproductive health, a young soon-to-be-married (and presumably virgin) woman was examined so that a (man) physician could "gently" instruct her about heterosexual penetrative sex in preparation for her wedding night. Such instruction involved both verbal remarks about sexuality and reproduction and vaginal penetration with a speculum to ensure that the bride-to-be was capable of having sex with her husband in this way. Influenced by Freudian theories of psychosexual development, physicians believed that a vaginal orgasm inside of marriage was the only form of healthy sexuality for adult women. By instructing women via the pelvic exam, physicians could therefore protect the sanctity of the (white, middle-class) nuclear family by ensuring a proper sexual order. These pronouncements were, of course, tied to racialized and heterosexist understandings of "normalcy": women of color and lesbians were discussed in the medical literature of this time only as pathological (Lewis 2005, 2010). In addition, while white women were "gently" instructed on proper womanhood including becoming mothers, poor women and women of color were targeted for coercive sterilization (Briggs 2003; López 2008; Roberts 1999). Thus, in this way, the pelvic exam has come to serve as a routine medical technology that shapes the gendered and racialized experience of having a body coded as female.

It should not be a surprise, then, that the pelvic exam was taught in such a manner that dehumanized its patients. It was also imbued with the expectation that women deserved to be in pain or could tolerate it without complaint—while those who could not were considered psychologically abnormal. For example, a medical textbook commonly assigned in the 1970s "tells medical students that 'mature' women don't react to pain": if "she is not 'relaxed' during a pelvic examination with an 'unlubricated speculum,' she might also be referred to a psychiatrist" (Weiss 1975:24–25).[10] Writing from a different point of view in the mid-1970s, a woman physician noted of her experience in medical school: "Coupled with these slights to female patients in medical school . . . are the attitudes and assumptions about 'woman's place' that color the doctor-patient relation. . . . One lecturer said, 'The only significant difference between a woman and a cow is that a cow has more spigots'" (Howell 1974:305).

The subjects of medical students' first introduction on the pelvic exam reinforced these messages about gender, the body, and medical authority. Prior to the gynecological teaching associate model, medical students first learned how to perform a pelvic exam on clinic patients (sometimes under anesthesia), plastic models, sex workers, or cadavers (Godkins et al. 1974; Kapsalis 1997; Kretzschmar 1978). As former GTA Terri Kapsalis argues:

> By using anesthetized women, cadavers, or plastic models as pelvic exam subjects students are being taught that a model patient (or patient model) is one who is essentially unconscious or backstage to the performance of the pelvic exam; she should be numb to the exam, providing no feedback and offering no opinions. . . . Passive and powerless female patients are considered ideal "participants" in the learning process. In addition, students practicing on essentially silent and lifeless models are learning that the manual skills associated with completing a pelvic exam are more important than the fundamental skills needed to interact with the patient. (1997:66)

These observations highlight several aspects of the practice of teaching and learning the pelvic exam prior to the advent of GTA programs. The pelvic exam involved an affective engagement characterized by a distinct *lack* of caring by the physician for his patient. Caring about the population via cervical cancer screenings and the management of appropriate reproduction was considered sufficient. Little care was taken for the patient (or the physician's) experience of the exam. This reflected a wider affective economy in which care was valued according to paternalistic standards in medicine: physicians were encouraged to care about patients in the abstract but strongly discouraged from developing emotional attachments to any patient in particular. One was to care for one's patients as a father does his children: through the provision of mandates that were in their best interest.

This all changed with the advent of the Women's Health Movement in the 1960s and 1970s, when some activists no longer accepted the existing practices of reproductive healthcare. "The Women's Health Movement" is a label that has come to be used by scholars to describe multi-sited rebellion by activists with varying goals and orientations toward mainstream medicine (Davis 2007; Kline 2010; Morgen 2002; Ruzek and Becker 1999; Zimmerman 1987). GTA program coordinator Martha described the kind of caring relationship valued prior to the advent the Women's Health Movement and activists' effects on the pelvic exam:

> I'm from the era [when] women were examined like flat on their back with a drape over their knees, and it was thought that . . . neither of us will talk, or I'll ask you what you did on your last vacation because we're both kind of embarrassed . . . so let's just pretend it's not happening. And women were also patronized. . . . Pat them on the knee and say, "Oh, don't worry about a thing, dear, I'll take care of you." And so . . . the rebellion and the women's movement, women were taught . . . tear that drape off their knees and sit up and say, "Talk to me face to face!"

In this model, women were to be taken care *of*, not cared *for* by an authoritative physician.[11] As Martha describes, the very material and spatial arrangements—flat on her back, drape over her knees preventing eye contact—reinforced this relationship. Any emotions experienced on either side of the encounter were to be quashed immediately. But the rebellion of the Women's Health Movement challenged these practices and *at the same time* the (lack of) a caring affective engagement between physician and patient. The movement targeted the material and technical practice of the pelvic exam in order to rewrite the ways in which physicians and patients interacted.[12] In short, it focused on practices in order to transform how physicians cared for—and about—patients.

Feminist activists in the Women's Health Movement were able to take on reproductive healthcare due in part to the emergence of self-help clinics and collectives. In such spaces, activists practiced pelvic exams on themselves and on one another in an effort to pry the tools of reproductive healthcare out of the hands of physicians (Morgen 2002; Murphy 2004). Activists taught each other how to perform abortions and treat vaginal infections themselves. Armed with this knowledge, feminists turned to mainstream medicine and demanded that physicians learn "to treat her [the patient] as a human being and not as an object" (Norsigian 1975:6). They argued that how medical students learned the pelvic exam laid the groundwork for how they would later treat women (Kapsalis 1997; Kline 2010; Norsigian 1975; Weiss 1975). These pronouncements politicized the pelvic exam, made it a matter of biopolitical contention. For example, feminists claimed that the way the pelvic exam was taught was dehumanizing, as it is in the above example where a physician is to refer a woman to a psychiatrist if she complains about discomfort when an unlubricated speculum is inserted into her vagina. As we have seen, they also pointed to how learning the exam on a passive woman lying flat on her back reinforced the idea that women lack agency or should be made to feel vulnerable. Likewise, feminists argued that use of clinic patients taught medical students that especially poor women of color deserved less respect than other women—an argument linked to critiques in feminism and racial justice projects of coercive sterilization as an abuse of medical authority. Finally, feminists were critical of the hiring of sex workers and of the belief that only "that kind" of woman (sexually amoral, sexually saturated) would willingly let strangers examine her, as well as the assumption that sex workers would be passive and compliant. Feminists argued that such a practice reinforced masculinist ideas of women as docile sexual objects, lacking agency and available for their use and disposal.[13] It is important to note that these activists did not reject the need for pelvic exams. Instead, they appropriated the tools of biomedicine and reworked them to fit into feminist models of care being developed in self-help clinics.

Thus, prior to the 1970s, the pelvic exam was a routine form of medical surveillance that sought to manage the health of the population through cervical cancer screenings and the instruction of white middle-class women in their proper roles as wives and mothers. This made it (and still makes it) a form of biopolitical power targeted toward the gendered and racialized body. However, the way the pelvic exam is practiced has changed quite dramatically. No longer are patients always positioned completely flat on their back, for example, or patted on the knee and told they'll be taken care of by a man in a white coat. Nor do medical school lecturers routinely and openly compare women to cows and recommend forcing specula into (understandably) recalcitrant vaginas; rather, great care is often taken to emphasize the importance of the patient's physical comfort and emotions. This transformation occurred in part due to the efforts of feminist activists.

Initial Collaborations and the Rise of Simulation

In the 1970s, feminist activists and a handful of medical educators began to reconsider ways of teaching and learning the pelvic exam in medical schools. Within biomedicine, medical school faculty became critical of the current models of teaching for three main reasons (Kretzschmar 1978). First, they were exploitative of the patients involved since these exams were purely educational and not for the health benefit of the patient. Second, students were anxious and unable to communicate freely with the instructor because of the patient's presence. Third, the patient was not able to provide detailed feedback to the student as to whether the proper organs had been palpated (i.e., medically examined). These critics tended to align themselves with the growing field of medical education research, which at the time was beginning to consider and develop standardized tools for assessing medical student performance, a story I tell in chapter 2. While medical educators were increasingly critical of the pelvic exam, they were also confronted by challenges from the Women's Health Movement.

The Women's Community Health Center provides one of the most prominent examples of an early collaboration between feminists and medical educators. In 1975, feminist activists embarked on a new way of teaching the pelvic exam when they were approached by women medical students at Harvard Medical School (Bell 1979; Editorial Submission 1975; Kline 2010). This first protocol involved women serving as pelvic models while a physician taught the students. Although this was satisfactory to the physicians, the women volunteers felt that they were being exploited. In response, these women formed the Pelvic Teaching Program (PTP), which recruited community members to teach the pelvic exam. In this second protocol, two women paired up to teach the exam while the physician remained a silent observer. This was a more agreeable model to the feminist activists, but an article about this teaching protocol that was published in *HealthRight* generated controversy. On one hand, some feminists saw them as an empowering way to have women teach medical students, which would ultimately challenge the dehumanization of patients during the exam. On the other, some activists saw how easily these programs could be coopted and lose their radical potential. Such critics recognized the institutional power of biomedicine to absorb challenges to its financial and social interests. "Teaching medical students ways to improve the pelvic exam for women was taken by [physicians] as a technique of managing their 'patients'" (Bell 1979:14). In their concerns about cooptation, activists thus identified a key phenomenon that would shape whether and how feminist politics of care could be incorporated into teaching and learning the pelvic exam. It had to do with the ways in which members of the medical profession could use feminist practices to meet their own interests. As a result, the collective strongly encouraged other women not to participate in similar programs without the support of a feminist collective behind them. These concerns about cooptation foreshadowed how GTA programs would evolve during the 1980s and point directly to the argument I make in this book: attending to emotion by generating affects of care and empathy is a strategy developed by medical education for managing patients.

The Women's Community Health Center developed a third protocol in order to address concerns over cooptation and depoliticization. This new protocol included several changes that addressed "hierarchy, sexism, fragmentation of learning skills, profit, and division between provider and consumer" (Bell, 1979: 12). The changes included (1) limiting the sessions to only women participants (and thus excluding men) in order to foster reciprocal sharing and challenge sexism in medicine, (2) inviting other hospital personnel to challenge physicians' dominance and the gap between provider and patient, (3) continuing the sessions over three or four separate occasions to foster critical discussion, and (4) increasing the cost from $25–$50 per session to $750 for all four sessions. Even though the group was approached by multiple medical schools, the protocol was not adopted by any. The reasons provided to the PTP were that the program was too expensive and excluded men, who medical faculty felt were most in need of such training. Thus, feminists were able to bring their political practices into the medical school so long as they followed the rules of the game. When they attempted to challenge basic tenets of medical power, they were unsuccessful.

Feminists in the PTP blamed the failure of their new protocol on the rigidity of medicine while also identifying a key history that would, in other medical schools, be the link between feminist politics of care and medical education: that of simulation. The members of the PTP were unaware when they began working with Harvard Medical School about experiments at other medical schools that use trained laypeople, known as simulated patients, to teach and evaluate clinical skills (Bell 1979; Kline 2010). Simulated patients emerged at other medical schools as a tech- nology that that could effectively manage the threat posed by the Wom- en's Health Movement's politicization of the pelvic exam by enclosing feminist demands and techniques within a system of medical expertise. Through simulated patients, medical educators could turn the relational experience between a physician and a patient into a standardized, mea- surable object, a history I discuss in more depth in chapter 2. Thus, while the third protocol of the PTP "confronted basic power relations and cur- rent assumptions about the goals of medical education," other ways of crafting GTA programs "fell within the acceptable range of innovations, exemplified by the 'Simulated Patient' programs" (Bell 1979:12).

The use of simulation in medical education has a long history, dat- ing back to at least the mid-sixteenth century in Europe, where mid- wives practiced their delivery skills on a basket-work frame covered in oilskin (Buck 1991).[14] During the 1960s, physicians began experiment- ing with the use of live people to simulate clinical encounters (Barrows and Abrahamson 1964; Wallace 1997). Using simulated patients allowed medical students to come "close to the truth of an authentic clinical encounter . . . without actually being there" (Wallace 1997:6). This coin- cided with a shifting ethical terrain in the 1960s and 1970s, when issues regarding informed consent and the exploitation of patients in service of furthering medical knowledge came to the fore. The use of simulated patients offered one solution: "The student can experience and practice clinical medicine without jeopardizing the health or welfare of real, sick patients" (Wallace 1997:6).

During the 1960s and 1970s at the University of Iowa, Robert Kretzschmar and his colleagues began experimenting with different models of teaching the pelvic exam. Kretzschmar disliked plastic models because they "lack authenticity . . . compared to the student's first encounter with a live patient," but using a patient was problematic, too: the "patient was exploited by the teaching system, as student examinations . . . do not contribute to patient care" (1978:367). The traditional method of teaching also did not address the interpersonal skills involved in performing the exam. At first, Kretzschmar and his colleagues recruited a nurse so that their students could practice the pelvic exam on a live person. However, she provided minimal feedback and her face remained draped to protect her privacy. By the 1970s, Kretzschmar was inspired by work with simulated patients and started a pilot program to recruit women to simultaneously teach the exam and be pelvic models.

Kretzschmar attributed the success of his program to the type of women he hired to work. His group of GTAs were six young women recruited from his university who were all "working toward or have received advanced degrees in the behavioral sciences" (Kretzschmar 1978:368). This made them qualified teachers. In addition, all were involved in some fashion with feminist health activism. Kretzschmar described the activist orientation of these GTAs as important to the work since they were concerned with "learning what it is to be a woman, exploring her own anatomy and physiology, and coming to terms with her sexuality, her attitudes, and her role in life" (1978:369). Hence, these women were comfortable with teaching and talking about the exam. In addition, Kretzschmar believed that these GTAs added "sensitivity and humanism" (1978:369) to the encounter. In this way, Kretzschmar used simulation as a technology that could both meet the needs of medical education *and* enfold some of the feminist practices of care into the pelvic exam. As he noted, "Rather than applying their skills elsewhere, whether it be through free medical clinics of women's health centers, the [GTAs] prefer to work within the existing system" (Kretzschmar 1978:368). By emphasizing the importance of these women's involvement in feminist health activism,

Kretzschmar seems to suggest that their politicization of the pelvic exam makes them amenable to reshaping the practice of the pelvic exam *within* the existing biomedical establishment. Unlike the PTP, Kretzschmar's program fit neatly into the "range of acceptable innovations" that Susan Bell (1979) criticized in her write up of the third protocol. This distinction also highlights the diversity of positions in the Women's Health Movement and their orientation toward biomedicine: some were cautiously optimistic about what they might be able to change in medical practice while others took a firmly antiestablishment approach.[15]

Thus, feminists were able to politicize the pelvic exam during the 1970s, but they were unable to sufficiently challenge the core tenets of biomedicine. Their concerns about how medical students learned the pelvic exam became assembled with medical educators' concerns as the practice of the pelvic exam passed out into the Women's Health Movement and back into medical schools. The key practice that allowed for this assemblage was simulation. As Adele Clarke and Joan Fujimura (2014) have shown, medical technologies must be made and "tinkered with" to make them into the "right tool" for the job. Technologies are adopted and modified by expert actors in order to make them into solutions for problems, which are themselves produced by social actors. Simulation emerged as the "right tool" for teaching and learning the pelvic exam through the actions of medical educators appropriating some aspects of feminist activism. Simulation is produced through expert discourses and practices. Its effects can be quantified and measured. Furthermore, simulation emerged as the right tool for the job because it could be made to capture the unruly forces of affect at work in teaching and learning the pelvic exam—for medical students, faculty, and patients. Put another way, through simulation, feminist practices of care could be brought into biomedicine without directly challenging its political and economic power.

Reassembling the Pelvic Exam at the University of Illinois at Chicago

I turn now to a case study to explore how the pelvic exam was reassembled during the 1980s out of interactions between feminist activists and researchers in medical education. The process of reshaping how medical students learned the pelvic exam reassembled bodies, affects, subjectivities, interactions between physician and patient, disciplinary practices, and professional social behaviors. I focus on the University of Illinois at Chicago (UIC) for three key reasons. First, the development of the GTA program at UIC is richly documented through scholarly publications and private archives. The program is quite representative of the processes and factors that led to the widespread creation and adoption of GTA programs. Second, UIC is home to one of the oldest, most well-established, and most influential centers devoted to medical education research: the Department of Medical Education. As such, it was where many of the key figures publishing the earliest accounts of GTAs came from. Third, Chicago was home to a prominent community of feminist health activists. The underground abortion network Jane was based in Chicago before *Roe v. Wade* legalized abortion access. The Emma Goldman Health Center—which is a key site in the story I tell here—was a flourishing women's self-help clinic that sought to raise women's consciousness about their health and bodies.

The first incarnation of the GTA program at UIC came at the very beginning of the 1980s when a group of medical students approached the Emma Goldman Health Center to prepare a workshop on the pelvic exam. It is significant that medical students themselves—rather than medical educators—first demanded change. According to my interviews, the impetus for the programs at two of the three medical schools I studied was a woman medical student.[16] This was at a time when large numbers of women were entering medical schools: whereas women made up 9.6 percent of medical students in 1970, the figures rose to 20.5 percent in 1976, 26.5 percent in 1981, and 32.5 percent in 1985 (AAMC 2016). Such a major demographic shift created instability in medical education, as women had begun to question the "boys in white" culture of medicine. In addition, while the widespread Vietnam War era protest of the 1960s had dissipated (Altbach and Cohen 1990), its effects lingered in medical schools. Commentators remarked on the change in the medical student body in the 1970s and 1980s, as students became more skeptical of the status quo and demanded more intensive socialization (Ebert 1986; Fox 1979).

Sally, one member of the group at UIC, described her motivation for seeking out help from the Emma Goldman Health Center:

> There was a . . . limited national movement . . . on the part of medical students in response to the Women's Healthcare Movement . . . to train more sympathetic, knowledgeable, and sensitive healthcare providers. So it was really a feminist sensibility of trying to train more appropriate healthcare providers that led [us] to emulate what was happening at a couple of medical schools in the country.

According to Sally, the students had learned about these other schools through student meetings at AAMC conferences. A volunteer from the Emma Goldman Health Center talked to the students about "the impact of the exam and how to do it in a thoughtful [manner], and then she allowed us to perform an exam and gave us feedback." The funds for this program came from the students involved. The source material—the "how to" of the pelvic exam—came from the Emma Goldman Health Center and feminist practices such as self-exam. It included more than just the actual mechanics of the exam: it also stressed how to talk to a patient and appreciate the patient's perspective during the exam, which is an affective component of care that became important to the later program.

However, this initial pairing of medical students with the Emma Goldman Health Center demonstrates some tensions that would run through the program. As historian Wendy Kline (2010) shows, there were longstanding political tensions among feminists due to differences in their orientation toward institutions. Members of the Emma Goldman Health Center originally took an oppositional stance toward the institution of medicine and refused to cooperate with physicians. More mainstream liberal feminist organizations such as the Chicago Women's Health Center and Planned Parenthood (the latter of which would provide activists for GTA training later on in the 1980s) were more amenable; in fact, according to Kline, as the Emma Goldman Health Center faced financial and staffing challenges, its members increasingly worked with the Chicago Women's Health Center and "even a group of young feminist OB-GYNs" (2010:82) at a nearby hospital. This also had effects on the racial politics of the program. Given how diverse and historically segregated Chicago is, Kline's analysis demonstrates that centers that did not explicitly center race in their missions tended to serve the interests of white women. This is significant because, while consciousness-raising groups were internally homogenous (Murphy 2012), self-help gynecology was not specifically the domain of white women (Morgen 2002; Nelson 2011). Self-help gynecology and self-exams were also important for Black Panther health activism and their community clinics (Nelson 2011). One activist, Norma Armour, even detected cervical cancer by performing her own Pap smear. However, while Black Panther community health clinics invited the flow of experts and tools *out* of biomedicine, they focused more on radically transforming structures of care, rather than on working within institutions to move experts and tools back *in* to biomedicine. For women in the UIC GTA program, working with and within institutions formed a more central component of their activism. I have no reliable data on the racial makeup of this group, but all of the members I was able to interview are white women. Efforts to recruit more women of color were unsuccessful, a topic I return to this issue later in the chapter.

The first workshop at UIC was only for the students who organized it, but eventually the students approached the administration and asked to make their program part of the curriculum. Sally was also pursuing a master's degree in Public Health at the time and decided to compare students who had gone through the program to those who had not in order to determine the program's impact. According to Sally: "That's the data that we used actually to propose this curricular change to . . . the medical school powers that be" and show that the program "would produce more capable and competent clinicians." The school ultimately accepted the proposal. Sally described students' initial reaction to the program as positive: "Most medical students were incredibly supportive and happy to have it because it really reduced the anxiety of doing your first pelvic exam." In this way, the feminist goal of caring for patients by making them feel comfortable aligned with the goal in medical education of reducing medical students' anxieties in order to foster their ability to learn.

Another important figure in the development of the program at UIC was MD physician Charles R. B. Beckmann. After a varied educational career, Charles chose a surgical specialty but quickly discovered that he preferred patient care: "I think that a key piece of medicine is hearing the patient and gaining the patient's trust. [For me, medicine is] not the money or prestige. It's about the joy of taking care of patients." One of Charles's earliest driving concerns was the importance of taking a good clinical history from a patient in order to direct the physical exam. As a gynecologist, his focus became the pelvic exam.

> It was a skill that if I watched people do it . . . I discerned a tremendous difference in the way they did it and the kind of information they got back. . . . And it had to do with, one, how they did it physically, and two, how they communicated, the level of trust the patient had, the patient being able to relax.

It is this observation that runs through the development of the program at UIC: the connection between style of practice and achieving the desired result. This observation also demonstrates an assemblage between the goal of making patients feel comfortable and empowered, as championed by the Women's Health Movement, and the goal in biomedicine of locating the truth of disease in the body through examination. Cultivating an affective stance of care toward the patient that would evoke trust, and thus relaxation, and would allow a physician to better find pathology on the patient's body. Charles's work then was central to plucking out from feminist politics the aspects of care that could be reassembled into the pelvic exam without challenging the core tenets of biomedicine.

Charles had a colleague who was running a GTA program at another university. This colleague introduced Charles to the GTAs and Charles spent time talking with them to learn about their motivations, their working conditions, and the ways they taught the exam. Interestingly, he also asked them their perspectives of gynecologists. In our interviews, Charles expressed an interest in finding out from the GTAs he worked with why women might dislike or distrust gynecologists so that his protocol for teaching the pelvic exam could correct these issues. He wanted to make physicians into likeable and trustworthy service providers. As he worked on the GTA program, Charles began to understand its implications for how medical students learned to build relationships with their patients. "I came to think that the . . . GTA session taught more about things that were happening outside of the pelvic [exam] than . . . inside the pelvic [exam]: . . . respect the patient, real understanding of partnership, real understanding of trust." While Charles's personal goals aligned with creating a better experience for patients by making providers more trustworthy, these efforts mapped onto larger challenges for the medical profession posed by the Women's Health Movement. Whether intentionally or not, creating more likeable physicians allowed the medical profession to re-secure its authority over reproductive healthcare.[17]

The timeline and exact process of how this happened is unclear, but at some point before or after his visit to his colleague's program, Charles became aware of what the medical students at UIC were doing. Charles himself doesn't remember how he became aware of it. According to Sally, Charles took over the program while she ran it as a resident under his authority. I suspect that Charles's identity as an experienced physician and a man lent more credibility to the program than Sally, who, as in many similar cases, received no formal credit for her contributions to the program. Her name appears nowhere in the publications of this time, although there is an obscure reference to the "programme founder" or "doctor founder" (Beckmann et al. 1988:125) interviewing potential GTAs in a published article.

With support from the chair of the Department of Obstetrics and Gynecology, Charles continued the program, working with Sally and an expanding group of GTAs drawn from the medical students' original workshop and their peer networks. The GTAs, "ordinary citizen with special knowledge and expertise" (Beckmann et al. 1988:128), were hired as contracted instructors. Charles's involvement in the program at this critical moment highlights the omnivorous ability of biomedical knowledge to absorb and refashion challenges to it. As the GTA program moved away from the early feminists' control and more into the control of medical education, its politics changed. For example, among the qualities that Charles looked for in potential GTAs were: "normal anatomy and the ability to relax sufficiently to allow easy examination . . . high intelligence, good verbal skills, commitment to better instruction for medical students and doctors in these skills, and personal maturity and emotional stability" (1988:125). The emphasis on normal anatomy and emotional stability is particularly evocative, given the gendered and racialized ways in which medical discourse constructs the female body in the pelvic exam. Normal anatomy meant that the body of the GTA had to mirror what medical students would learn from the anatomical atlas, while emotional stability raises the specter of the hysterical woman whose body is "thoroughly saturated with sexuality" (Foucault 1990:104).

The initial protocol was developed out of conversations among Charles and the GTAs: "Many, many, many hours sitting together talking about their experiences, frustrations, their experiences with friends and what they thought was wrong, what they thought was right." Charles cites as an example what had been a common practice of calling the woman patient a pet name like "honey" or "sweetie": "It was taught in many places that was a way to help a woman relax. Well, it's just the opposite for most women. And it certainly is degrading. [To] a man you wouldn't say, 'Honey, bend over. I want to stick my finger up your butt.'" The GTAs in this early program motivated Charles to address these commonplace practices that resulted in such demeaning experiences. This linked up with Charles's professed interest in understanding how style of practice was related to health-related outcomes such as being able to identify early signs of pathology. And certainly, such a culture of casual sexism contributed to women seeking out alternatives to mainstream biomedicine. By addressing practices that drove women away, medical educators like Charles could reestablish medical authority. In this way, women's feelings about the exam and about physicians had to be addressed and modulated through new types of expert practices.

This goal mapped on to those that feminists also held. Ruth, who had been a GTA at the time, told me, "I really wanted to get into the eye of the storm, to train these motherfuckers [*laughs*] on how to do this right and how to get the information that they needed from their patients so that they could formulate the proper care diagnosis." Likewise, Jaclyn said:

> I hope in some ways it was a humbling experience . . . [to] counter some of the . . . arrogance that medical students . . . are . . . trained to have. I don't believe they come in to school with that. . . . They were . . . trained to have a certain degree of authority and that somehow authority leads to good healing. . . . I think the experience of having somebody who you're examining . . . in a very kind of intense way . . . hopefully opened them up to the idea that that these were people with knowledge and experiences

and things that they could potentially learn from. . . . And hopefully it would lead to more respect and closer communication with their patients.

A few other GTAs who were working in the early to mid-1980s echoed a similar sentiment about their motivation for doing the work. Early GTAs like Ruth and Jaclyn felt that training better physicians would improve reproductive healthcare in the long run.

Publications about the program from this time emphasize the feminist orientation of the GTAs and espoused it importance for the program's success at achieving its goals (Beckmann et al. 1988:125). These women's comfort and experience allowed them, in Charles's view, to be ideal teachers and work well with students. He describes treating them as authorities regarding their own experiences: "They had a very strong sense of autonomy, which I . . . am sincerely supportive [of]." This once again highlights the kind of feminist activism that was involved in creating GTA programs:

> The [GTAs] are, in part, attracted to this ambiguous situation because they see it as a way of having positive influence on the training of doctors while not becoming incorporated within the medical education establishment which they may perceive as chauvinistic. The feminist orientation of the [GTA program] is thereby preserved without constraints imposed by the academic organization. (Beckmann et al. 1988:128).

Some feminists might be skeptical about the institution, but they were still willing to work within it to challenge the provision of reproductive healthcare.

The GTAs and Charles worked together on how to teach the skills of the pelvic exam to the medical students. One aspect of this preparation was a great deal of practice with the manual aspect of the exam, especially the speculum insertion, so that the GTAs could develop embodied knowledge about what a proper exam felt like. "And so one of the things we practiced is the women doing the teaching knowing what it felt like to have the speculum not far enough in and far enough in." What Charles learned from these practice sessions with the GTAs ultimately went into his textbook on the exam: "We learned a lot about how does it [the speculum] fit? Not just the obvious things, like warming the speculum, picking the right size speculum. . . . You need to be careful that you insert the speculum at the right angle. . . . It's not perpendicular to the floor, but it's tilted upward slightly." This contrasts starkly with previous techniques for performing the pelvic exam, in which a patient who complains about the speculum insertion is to be referred to a psychiatrist. What is striking about these techniques as well is that they are taken almost directly from the Women's Health Movement. A 1976 document from the Women's Community Health Center, "How to Do a Pelvic Examination," describes exactly the same method for inserting a speculum.

Similarly, Charles learned to be mindful of the appropriate angles when performing the rectovaginal exam, which involves inserting the middle finger into the rectum and the index finger into the vagina to examine the tissue between rectum and vagina. Rather than inserting the fingers straight on, he and the GTAs discovered that a horse-shoe shaped motion was more comfortable. Charles and the GTAs learned about physical stance for performing the bimanual exam, which involves inserting two fingers into the vagina to examine the cervix, uterus, and ovaries. Standing too close or too far away makes the exam difficult and emotionally uncomfortable for the patient, while tucking the elbow at the side and extending through the wrist makes it more physically comfortable for the physician and allows for better leverage.

The GTAs were encouraged to adjust the speculum in the teaching encounter so that students would learn how to properly insert it. They learned to pair this instruction on exam skills with instruction on proper communication, all with the goal of reducing student anxiety to make the exam a better experience for patients. Charles explained: "The teaching wasn't just the exam, but they [would] talk about how they [the students] were feeling and . . . if you make a mistake don't worry about it. We're trained so well . . . you can't hurt us." Thus, reassembling the exam was not only about developing manual or technical practice. It was also about acknowledging medical students' own emotional states, so that they could be examined and set aside or cultivated appropriately for professional practice. Anxiety in particular had to be managed so that medical students could appear to be confident and composed for the patient's sake, no matter how they actually felt. In this way, the GTA program also aligned with a larger movement in medical education at the time to redefine professionalism to include acknowledgment and management of emotion, both patient and physician.[18]

The program demonstrated success. According to Charles, "The administration liked the way the students came out, liked the way they felt about themselves, what they perceived their skills to be and the feedback from [their preceptors] was they're better at it." However, Charles experienced resistance from "the family doctors, some of the internists and others": "They were terrified there were going to be affairs, there was going to be sexual activity." Some faculty members expressed concerns that paying women to receive pelvic exams was unethical and akin to prostitution. Their concerns echo those expressed in some of the literature at the time, that no "normal" woman would allow herself to be examined by strangers in this manner (Kapsalis 1997). Indeed, scholars of the pedagogical practice of the pelvic exam have pointed out the tenuous borders between shame and pleasure that exist when a person's vagina is put on display in this way (Bell 2009). Charles defended his GTAs as being skilled educators—as they were: these early GTAs developed a unique stock of bodily knowledge that qualified them as experts. The systematic valuing of GTAs' bodily knowledge as the program became more institutionalized challenged what could count as expertise in medical education. This reassembled what kinds of knowledge counted as legitimate in biomedicine and who might be authorized to teach this knowledge to neophytes in the profession.

Working together, Charles and these early GTAs dismantled, interrogated, and refashioned multiple elements of the pelvic exam. GTAs practiced insertion techniques and the bimanual exam on one another in order to learn how to teach it. In the process, Charles learned about more appropriate and more comfortable techniques, which he incorporated into the protocol. Thus, *the manual and technical technique* of the pelvic exam was reassembled through the development of the GTA program. Charles and the GTAs also focused on language and communication during the exam, removing words and phrases that were sexist, demeaning, or otherwise offensive. They incorporated ways to inform the patient about the exam as it was being performed, such as showing the patient the speculum and explaining its purpose. In this way, not only was the *language of the pelvic exam* reassembled, but the *relationship between physician and patient* was reassembled as well. The docile patient was replaced with a more informed one. Finally, by focusing on the feelings of the medical students and by talking about how sensitive and sexually charged this exam can be, Charles and the GTAs he worked with were attempting to change medical students' own perceptions and attitudes toward learning the pelvic exam so that they felt safe acknowledging their embarrassment, discomfort, and fear of failure or hurting the patient. The *affect of the medical student* was reassembled. These changes were all related to critiques that feminist activists had of teaching and learning the pelvic exam, and many of these techniques came from the GTAs' experiences working in feminist self-help. In this way, feminists were able to bring some of the movement's practices of care into medical education.

What is a "Good" Pelvic Exam? The Development of the Protocol

During the late 1980s, as medical education developed a distinct regime of expertise, the GTA session was shaped by standardizing and institutionalizing forces. This occurred at the national level and played out on the ground at UIC. As the GTA program at UIC developed, two faculty members in the Office of Research in Medical Education were brought in to evaluate it. Their involvement came as the program had become somewhat established and attention shifted toward standardizing the curriculum. A key technology in this process was the communication checklist, which is a standardized method of teaching and assessing physician-patient interaction skills.

Elaine, a faculty member with a sciences PhD, adapted her work on such a checklist for the GTA program: "So in the checklist was . . . how you introduce yourself to the patient, how you approach the patient with comfort and modesty and all those things. . . . The GTAs were told about the expectations for . . . what a good exam would be so that they would know what to provide feedback." The GTAs were given this checklist in order to adapt their teaching styles to it and to use it in evaluating each medical student at the end of the session. The goal of standardizing the curriculum was twofold: it made certain that medical students were being taught *and* evaluated consistently, according to Elaine:

Having a standardized checklist [is important] so that you could get some consistency. . . . The ability to say, okay, this is what we all agree on as a good exam . . . here is what the steps should look like . . . so that when their students are evaluated, they're all evaluated according to the same criteria.

Thus, developing a protocol that could be consistently taught to all medical students *and* used to evaluate them meant a certain amount of durability and concretizing of what officially counts as a good pelvic exam through the GTA session. This brought feminist politicization into clinical practice as a matter of best practices in medical education. Many of the tenets of feminist practice became cornerstones of the checklist: respecting the patient's bodily autonomy, actively involving the patient in the exam, and using language that was not derogatory or distancing (for examples of these checklists, see appendix B). Moreover, these tenets remain fundamental in GTA programs across the United States. My interviews with current and former GTAs reveal that the curriculum has remained largely unchanged since the late 1980s or early 1990s when the checklist was adopted. However, standardizing the protocol had consequences for how explicitly political the program could be.

Nancy, a faculty member with a social sciences PhD, also worked on the checklist. She identified another area of concern for the program.

We had problems . . . in trying to diversify along racial and ethnic lines. The women for the program . . . were . . . mainly white women, and we had a little bit of diversity but we found it difficult to get the kind of diversity . . . that would really represent the patient population at [the] hospital.

Given the recruitment strategies for GTAs—coming through feminist organizations and word-of-mouth—the internal composition of the group was fairly homogenous. According to Nancy, faculty members "tried to do outreach to different communities and so forth," including reaching out to a Latina feminist organization, but ran into challenges. In our interview, Nancy cites "cultural taboos" on receiving pelvic exams from men physicians as a reason, alongside the internal homogeneity of GTAs' social groups. She identified the racial politics of different feminist orientations toward working in or against institutions that I discussed earlier: "The women that were most motivated because they wanted to improve women's health tended to be white, probably well-educated women." Changes within the program to emphasize the professionalization of GTAs also likely exacerbated these challenges.

According to Donna, a GTA during the late 1980s: "There was a real push to, you know, make the whole thing more professional, to bring it up to a certain level." The GTAs working at the time were used to a more relaxed style of practice that was common in feminist self-help circles. Tardiness and flexibility of work schedules, as well as wearing casual clothing, had been typical for the GTAs. Then the coordinator insisted that GTAs show up to work on time and begin to dress more professionally (which meant no ripped or dirty clothing, which mattered at the time because GTAs first greeted their students fully clothed before stepping out to change into a hospital gown). This coordinator also began to more heavily emphasize offering constructive criticism to students and adhering to the standardized curriculum that had been developed, rather than going "off script" by talking about whatever the GTA felt was important. This push to "make the whole thing more professional" signaled a radical shift in the GTA program. As it became more subsumed under medical education, its earlier elements of feminist rebellion had to be shaken off. This created a great deal of political tension in the program.

Around this time, this coordinator left and was replaced by another coordinator who was even more insistent on adhering to these changes. It is unclear whether this shift was intentional or the result of individual preferences on the part of the new coordinator, who had also been a GTA. She refused to allow GTAs to discuss topics such as abortion rights and access to contraceptives, which she thought were too political. In addition, she disallowed GTAs from teaching while menstruating. The coordinator, whom I interviewed, felt that medical students were already nervous enough and confronting a menstruating body would make the encounter too anxiety-provoking, thus inhibiting their ability to learn. This prohibition became a politically charged issue for some of the GTAs. Sylvia told me:

> There was one coordinator that I just would not work with . . . because she would not allow GTAs to work if they were menstruating . . . she just

had a very medical approach. . . . She would come back during the training sessions for us and report that, oh, a student had said that we were too
feminist. . . . She just didn't come from the women's health perspective.

For these GTAs, menstruation was a natural function of the body and
teaching while menstruating was important in order to foster that recognition and its value in medical students. Most GTAs preferred not
to teach while menstruating, as it could be messy and uncomfortable
for them.[19] However, being prohibited from teaching while menstruating became, for some GTAs, an issue of political concern, as it removed
the choice from the individual GTA and made it a policy of the GTA
program.

These contestations intensified as the program shifted more fully
away from feminist control and into medical education, since practices
had to align with the standards and values of the institution. Coordinators began to emphasize supporting students' education over espousing
feminist politics of care. According to Jaclyn, a GTA at this time, "It went
from there being a coordinator who felt like she was coming at it partly
from an activist position to a coordinator who was much more about . . .
we're tools of the institution and we need to do everything exactly how
they say and that's how it needs to be done." This led to a crisis within the
GTA working group about the politics of the program and who really
controlled the curriculum. Sylvia told me:

> It was outrageous and I really thought that . . . we really needed to union-
> ize and really become more professional in our own right . . . so that
> we could be stronger in terms of the curriculum and the education
> program. . . . We essentially had no control over that. We had control over
> what we did in the room once the students got there, but no control
> over what . . . they had been told before they came into the room.

Sylvia and GTAs like her echoed the feminist politics of the 1970s, drawing on socialist feminist notions of workers' rights to describe their
work. The GTAs who espoused this position seem to have been mainly
those who had come to the program through the Emma Goldman
Health Center and had worked with the original group of medical students. The GTAs who had come from a network of activists working at

Planned Parenthood were less outraged by the prohibition. Donna, who came in through a friend just a little bit after Sylvia, gave a slightly different account of the situation:

> They wanted to own the program . . . They were invited in by the medical students, but it . . . became so successful . . . the Emma Goldman people decided that—they went after [Charles]. Some of them didn't like him and they thought that he was, you know, anti-feminist or something weird like that. . . . They tried to like get everybody to go on strike and not go to work. And the thing was that it paid so well that . . . most of the women that were doing it were doing it for the pay and not for a political purpose anymore.

The language of unionization and going on strike speaks directly to feminist politics of the 1970s. Campaigns such as Wages for Housework mobilized strikes and anti-work tactics to underscore women's reproductive labor (Cox and Federici 1976; Weeks 2011). Likewise, sex workers have also used strikes as tactics (Smith and Mac 2018). However, according to Donna and Sylvia, this attempted reassertion of power ultimately backfired, and the GTAs who had supported it chose to leave the program. The GTA program had become too depoliticized to make these tactics successful. Explicit feminist politics were no longer welcome.[20]

While many GTAs nationwide continue to actively maintain a feminist orientation to their work, some of the Chicago-area GTAs who have been working since the 1980s expressed to me, either formally or informally, frustration with a loss of politics from the program. Emphasizing the history of the physician-patient relationship and training medical students to respect their patients has been deemphasized in favor of making the encounter more about reducing the anxiety of medical students. GTA Vivian told me, "As it's [the GTA program] evolved, I think less and less of [the] feminist movement of, you know, address me as an equal. It's not about that. It's about the anatomy. It's not about being respected as a female. I think that's a forgone conclusion at this point." This transformation is part of the broader shift in the affective economy of medical education as faculty have begun to differently value the emotional experiences of students. According to Martha, a program coordinator:

Medical student started having groups where they actually talked about how they felt about cutting up dead bodies and . . . things changed, sort of like the women's movement, you know. We no longer have to fight so hard, I think, and some things are just accepted and taken for-granted and part of this society. And so then it became more about just how to make it a more comfortable experience . . . for the women you're examining.

Sally, the medical student who helped found the GTA program at UIC, reflected:

I think the historical underpinnings of a feminist basis for it are completely lost. I think now it's just all about education. And that's not wrong. But I think there's something to be learned from a notion that, you know, the common perception was that we [physicians] were uncaring . . . and not thoughtful in [our] approach to how to conduct a reproductive health exam. So I think the program brought about a change in sensibility and cultural awareness.

According to Sally, the explicit feminism of the exam has been lost, but its aims were met by bringing about transformation in the way physicians relate to their patients and perform the pelvic exam. In this way, as feminist practices were brought into medical education, only some aspects of feminist care were palatable to the institution and to GTAs themselves. Making medical students more comfortable in order to improve their educational experience was acceptable, while confronting power relations and hierarchies in medicine was not.[21]

The result for teaching and learning the pelvic exam was a declining significance in the politics of care in US medical education. A number of forces that made affect a problem to be managed declined, and the rise of medical education as an academic discipline meant a form of expertise that could more effectively "govern at arms' length" (Rose 1993) through managing affect. The US Women's Health Movement has waned. At the same time, the gender composition of medical students has become more equal. By 1993, women made up 40 percent of medical students, and by 2005, 48.5 percent (AAMC 2016). During the 1990s, a number of courses and working groups were developed to address medical students' emotions in relationship to doing physical exams.

Consumerist pressures led to a radical transformation in professional practices, as clinical medicine moved from being physician-centered to patient-centered (Clarke et al. 2003; Laine and Davidoff 1996). The culture around informed consent and patients' rights changed with the emergence of biomedicalization: patients are more informed and proactive in general, and physicians are more mindful of the patient experience for a number of reasons. Thus, a new regime emerged as medicine developed expertise in managing the threat of affect more effectively.

Instrumentality and the Politics of Care

The standardization of the "good" pelvic exam in the GTA session mapped onto national-level transformations in medical education. As I discuss in the next chapter, the development of checklists and simulated patients aligned with the increasingly science-oriented nature of medicine. Charles and his colleagues gathered data on medical student performance and anxiety before and after the GTA session, and they published several articles in medical journals. Their research added to a growing body of literature on GTA programs, as these types of programs gained widespread acceptance. In 1985, 77 percent of medical schools in the United States and Canada used GTA programs (Beckmann et al. 1985). This number remained unchanged until 1992 (Beckmann et al. 1992). This diffusion of GTA programs into the routine practices of medical schools demonstrates both the institutionalization of these programs, which remains relatively unchanged today (Dugoff et al. 2016), and aligns with other analyses of how elements of the Women's Health Movement have been coopted by biomedicine (Ruzek and Becker 1999; Thomas and Zimmerman 2007).

The cooptation of feminist practices leads me back to a critical analysis of the politics of care present in the pelvic exam. Certainly, the pelvic exam has been reassembled in many key ways as feminist politics of care were appropriated by medical education. And yet, I "unsettle care" (Murphy 2015) to fully understand the ramifications. I believe it is possible to hold space for both the positive ways in which feminist principles of care have transformed the pelvic exam at the same time that I acknowledge the exclusions and limitations. While I will return to these tensions throughout the book as I discuss new strategies of governance in medical education that rely on the modification of affect, I highlight several of them now.

One tension involves the relationship between feminism and the economic interests of the medical profession. The Women's Health Movement and the growing number of alternatives to mainstream medicine, such as self-help clinics, provided a direct economic challenge to medicine (Thomas and Zimmerman 2007). This is related to a whole host of transformations in the political economy of health care at the same time, encapsulated by discussions of consumerism in medicine (Tomes 2016). Moreover, with a growing public distrust of experts of all kinds in the 1970s (Frickel and Moore 2006), medicine *had* to listen to the activists of the Women's Health Movement in order to get their share of the market back. In this way, the practices of care that feminists espoused were assembled into medicine under the wholesale shift from physician-centered to patient-centered practices. Physicians had to learn new ways to not just care for but also care *about* patients as patients increasingly shopped around for their healthcare. In this configuration of the politics of care, the cooptation of feminist practices of care have made the exercise of medical authority more palatable to patients *in order to* bolster the economic interests of medicine (Vinson 2016). Two excellent examples of this development come from Charles's observation that style of practice in the pelvic exam was linked to the kind of information that a physician could get back from a patient and his conversations with GTAs about what exactly women did not like about gynecologists. In this way, medical education research was able to render feminist practices of care into techniques for assuring the trust and compliance of patients.

A second tension involves how feminist practices of care have translated into research on medical education. Affect must be translated from experience into language in order to be knowable to science. In a similar way, because the use of simulation allowed medical education to coopt feminist practices of care, these practices had to be rendered into something standardized, objective, and measurable. Feminist self-help was especially amenable to this kind of cooptation because it had politicized the technical details of the pelvic exam. This occurred at the same time as a movement in medical education toward standardized evaluations of medical student performance (rather than just knowledge). Feminist practices of care that could be distilled down to measurable behaviors could be incorporated into teaching and learning the pelvic exam, while those that were more relational or that targeted structures of healthcare (such as access or control) could not and were left by the wayside. This is evident in the first checklists: behaviors and attitudes could be incorporated, while innovations such as the Pelvic Teaching Program's third protocol could not. What could be standardized could be coopted.

A third tension centers on who is being cared *for* in teaching and learning the pelvic exam. Ostensibly, the GTA program arose in response to medical mistreatment of patients. And yet, as the program continued, it lost its political teeth. It became much more of a program about tending to the emotional experiences of medical students. This is evident in Ruth's language about getting into "the eye of the storm" and teaching "these motherfuckers" the right way to treat women and Jaclyn's concerns about becoming "tools of the institution." Feminist practices of care are very much about relationality and extending empathy and compassion to both participants in the pelvic exam. As the program was distilled down to checklists and measurements, the care for the patient that had animated GTAs' work mutated into caring for medical students. This is not to say that medicine should revive its old practices of crushing the emotional experiences of medical students under the cultural mandate of detached concern. Rather, it is to invoke concern for the gendered nature of this work. The emergence of feminist practices of care were tied to critiques about the devaluing of feminized labor. And while GTAs have been able to stake a claim for compensation for their bodily knowledge, there is something notable about the labor they perform of *taking care of* medical students during this emotionally fraught encounter. This underscores how the work that GTAs do involves a great deal of emotional labor, which I discuss in chapters 3 and 4.

Fourth, and finally, the practices of care ultimately adopted in teaching and learning the pelvic exam attended to the concerns of some types of people and not others. The kinds of feminist ideologies that found working within institutions acceptable tended to center the concerns of women who were willing and able to submit themselves to medical authority as part of the yearly pelvic exam. Their politics of care did not encompass questions of access or the racialized politics of coercive sterilization. When feminists and other radical health activists did

challenge the capitalist and white supremacist underpinnings of reproductive healthcare, they were locked out of the institution or else chose
to work elsewhere to expand access and knowledge to the communities most affected. The consequences of this kind of political and ideological division meant that only forms of feminist protest that aligned
with the larger goals of biomedicine were coopted. As a result, teaching
and learning the pelvic exam follows along the lines of the immediate
concerns of making patients comfortable and compliant with medical
authority.

I am deeply critical here of how care has been rendered instrumental:
practices of care have become in their own way a kind of technology
of affect in the pelvic exam. Yes, patients are cared *about* now, not just
cared *for*, and yet these forms of care are uneven in their application and
in their effects. I will never want us to return to the days when a woman
is selected from a clinic to become an "anonymous vagina" to be probed
by novice medical students, but I am also concerned by the ways that
making the pelvic exam less frightening are entangled with capitalism
and medical authority. I argue that medical education is increasingly
organized around technologies of affect and forms of affective governance that seek to harness, modify, and, ultimately, make profit out of
embodied capacities to feel. I consider more fully how simulation is a
key technology of affect in this new regime in the next chapter.

2

From Assessing Knowledge to Assessing Performance

GTA Programs, Medical Education Research,
and Technologies of Affect

A pelvic examination does not have to be a traumatic
experience for either the woman being examined or the
examiner. Your own attitude can make a profound difference
when you do a pelvic. If you are relaxed, you are less likely
to make the woman nervous. If you are interested in teaching the woman about her body, if you can give reassurance
and positive feedback . . . and especially if you explain what
you are doing and why as you go along, the woman will feel
more comfortable herself with the procedure. You will both
be learning, which, in turn, facilitates better health care.
—How to Do a Pelvic Examination, Women's Community
Health Center, 1976

The interaction during a pelvic examination can be divided
into those behaviors which are solely the responsibility of
the doctor, including verbal and nonverbal behavior, and
those which require active participation of the patient. . . .
Attention to all types of interaction sets a climate to
facilitate a quality pelvic exam.
—Pelvic Examination Instruction, Ms. Reiter, Ms. Hamilton,
and Ms. Guenther, circa 1980

Checklists may be used for teaching and/or for assessment.
Grading may be by yes/no or expanded to include assessment of task completion to fully/partially/not done/not
applicable. The checklist should be completed by a trained
observer with knowledge of the proper technique of the
pelvic examination.
—The Pelvic Exam, Association of Professors of Gynecology
and Obstetrics, 2008

These are all examples of instructions for teaching and learning the pelvic exam at different historical moments in the development of gynecological teaching associate programs.[1] What is evident in how these instructions have evolved over time is that feminist practices of care have been coopted by medical education, a story that I tell in chapter 1. And yet, there is another story in them, one that links the growth and institutionalization of GTA programs with a broader trend in medical education. In all of these examples, there is a slightly different approach to how the GTA program that produced it conceptualizes the physician-patient relationship. It starts as an intersubjective phenomenon in which feelings circulate between physician and patient, becomes a set of skills both verbal and nonverbal, and morphs into an *object* that can be graded by an expert.

The first example was produced by the Pelvic Teaching Program, the feminist self-help organization that I discussed in the previous chapter. In these instructions, medical students should attend carefully to cultivating a relationship with the patient, one that benefits both the physician and the patient to the betterment of healthcare in general. The second was used to formulate the protocol at one of the GTA programs that I studied in Chicago (see appendix B). These instructions provide examples of verbal and nonverbal behaviors as a numbered list, such as "Use supportive tone of voice" and "Use appropriate level of terminology." In this iteration, the physician-patient relationship has been distilled down to a set of behaviors that a trained observer such as a GTA can teach. The "reassurance and positive feedback" of the first set of instructions is more concretely identified as tone of voice, for example.

In the third example, a checklist produced by a national professional organization to be used by GTAs to formally evaluate students at the end of the session, students' verbal and nonverbal behaviors are given in a table format (see appendix B).[2] Down the rows are phrases such as "Uses appropriate eye contact, body language," "Uses facilitative listening skills," "Demonstrates empathy," and "Attends to patient's comfort." Across the columns are labels: "Well Done," "Needs Improvement," "Not Done," and "Cannot Recall." In this most recent iteration, the relationship between a physician and patient has been assembled into a table so that its components can be checked off alongside behaviors such as washing one's hands and securing the speculum in an open position. In short, what has happened is a wholesale shift toward capturing the physician-patient relationship through this kind of standardization of the observable and demonstrable behaviors associated with "good" professional practice.

GTA programs arose during the 1980s as medical schools were reconsidering whether merely evaluating a students' *knowledge* was sufficient or whether students' *performance* should also be evaluated.[3] In this chapter, I am concerned with how this shift has produced the relationship between a physician and patient in the pelvic exam, treated as an object of expert concern. Indeed, as I have shown already, major transformations in the economic, social, and political organization of medicine during the 1970s and 1980s reshaped the expectations for how a physician would relate to a patient. And yet, what I have not explored is the larger apparatus of expert knowledge that enabled medical education to respond to these changes and reassert the professional dominance of medicine. This move included the formation of new sets of knowledges and practices that could deploy expertise over how best to produce the next generation of physicians. As research on best practices proliferated, what was inherently subjective—the relationship between a physician and patient—became something possible to assess objectively and empirically—by checklist, by survey, by written examination.[4] This occurred through the codification of an academic discipline devoted to research on medical education.

I argue that GTA programs are part of a larger trend in which medical education expanded its control over the professional socialization of medical students through an increasing array of knowledges and practices—which I call *technologies of affect*—that seek to measure, harness, and manage the affective capacities of medical students. As the affective economies of healthcare shifted, new forms of governance via expert knowledges and technologies were necessary in order to prepare physicians-in-the-making for a changing landscape of clinical practice in which emotion figures centrally. These technologies seek to discipline affect in order to produce medical experts who can more effectively govern the conduct of their patients. Indeed, the reconfiguration of expertise and affect via research on medical education is highly evident in the GTA session *and* explains its durability and relevance.

In this chapter I trace the growth of research on simulated patients and the communication and interpersonal skills checklist. GTAs are a subset of simulated patients whose work has been standardized by this kind of checklist, as I discuss in chapter 1. Simulated patients and communication and interpersonal skills checklists are technologies produced by medical education research, an academic discipline that takes as its object the best ways to produce physicians as qualified experts in a particular economic, social, and political climate. While others have told the history of medical education research since its origins in the 1950s (Kuper, Albert, and Hodges 2010; Rangel et al. 2016), in this chapter I trace how and why medical education research rose to prominence as a guiding body of expertise and extended control over the affective capacities of medical students (and by extension patients), as well as look at the kinds of technologies it produces to discipline such capacities. Teaching and learning the pelvic exam are, again, my central example.

"What Can Be More Logical Than to Consult with Specialists?" Reconfiguring Expertise and Affect in Medical Education Research

I claim that medical education research represents a unique type of expertise that takes as its central question how best to produce and certify physicians. I am informed by debates in the literature on the move from thinking about experts as kinds of people produced in socially and culturally specific places to thinking about expertise as a system of knowledges and practices (Collins and Evans 2008; Evans 2008; Eyal 2013). Indeed, a "full explication of expertise must explore . . . this background of practices and the social, material, spatial, organizational, and conceptual arrangements that serve as its conditions of possibility" (Eyal 2013:871). Thus, framing medical education research through the lens of expertise allows me to examine the networks of practices and knowledges and the tools and devices (among which I consider technologies, in the Foucauldian sense) used to accomplish the task of educating the next generation of physicians. Separating medical expertise from medical education research throughout my analysis,[5] I show how the tools of science—in particular, the psy-sciences—merged with transformations in the affective economies of healthcare to shape the "conditions of possibility" (Eyal 2013:871) by which new physicians could be made and certified. In short, new tools, practices, and knowledges were necessary to grapple with new constellations of affect in clinical practice.

Medical education research as a distinct academic discipline began in the 1950s in the United States, alongside the shoring up of professional authority through the growth of science and technology.[6] During this formative period, medical educators increasingly turned to the tools of science as they determined best practices for educating the next generation of physicians. The debates—and the eventual solution discovered in the psy-sciences—set the stage for the kind of experimentation and research projects that physician-educators such as Robert Kretzschmar and Charles R. B. Beckmann would undertake in the 1970s and 1980s for new methods of teaching and learning the pelvic exam.

The earliest projects in medical education research emerged in the post–World War II period. This was a time of crisis and transformation in medicine and the medical profession, and it was also a time of growing interest in psychology as a scientific discipline (Orr 2006; Rose 1998). These changes altered the field of clinical practice and how medical students learned to become physicians. The amount of scientific and technological information that medical students were required to learn intensified, putting pressure on already full curricula. Medical school faculty and administers became concerned about admissions standards; schools needed to be admitting students who could keep up with the increasingly science-oriented materials (Kuper et al. 2010). In addition, public demands for accountability in the profession, coupled with public interest and demand for new science, put pressure on medical schools.

Because of these external pressures on the medical profession, medical faculty became interested in not only reforming their curricula, but also systematically understanding whether their changes had their intended effects. This meant using the tools of science, such as empirical research. A handful of medical schools developed interest in "comprehensive medicine," which was intended to reinvigorate medical students' concern for the patient at the heart of medical training by increasing attention to the psychological and social aspects of illness (Kendall and Reader 1988). Medical faculty began to evaluate such interventions through such practices as comparing an experimental group to a control group. In a piece in the *Journal of the American Medical Association*, one physician suggested that medical education should follow the principles of engineering: "the art of applying scientific knowledge to tasks of living" (Ross 1962:140). This led to a push toward formalization by scholars interested in researching medical education.[7]

Psychology was at the heart of these curricular experiments and the methods for evaluating their effectiveness. Educational psychology was thought to be particularly applicable to evaluating and improving curricula. This is evident in the first systematic evaluation of the preparedness of medical educators to teach students, which occurred at the University of Buffalo, New York, during the 1950s. Medical faculty member George Miller led these efforts.

> Coming from the world of medicine, where a physician seeks the aid of a specialist in those situations in which he feels such assistance is necessary, what could be more logical, Dr. Miller asked, than to consult with specialists in education when problems in instruction and evaluation arise? (Abrahamson 1960:38)

The Commonwealth Fund provided funds for a series of seminars over three years to introduce faculty of the University of Buffalo to a variety of educational techniques (Miller 1980). Although the project ultimately failed, the report the participants produced became the book *Teaching and Learning in Medical School*, published in 1961, which reexamined the process of teaching medical students. The *Journal of the American Medical Association* called it a "direct attack on insularly held cherished beliefs and practices rampant in our medical schools" (Miller 1980:77).

By 1961, three medical schools had official departments dedicated to research in medical education: Western Reserve (now Case Western Reserve University), the Medical College of Virginia, and the University of Illinois, whose significance in developing and systematically studying the GTA program I demonstrate in chapter 1 (Rosinski 1988). Other programs soon emerged, so that by the mid-1960s, there were seven offices of research in medical education nationally. The nascent discipline of medical education research thus had the beginnings of institutional support through the founding of such offices or departments within medical schools. Other signs of formalization included the publication of specialty journals,[8] as well as funding for systematic research in medical education made possible by three separate federal acts passed between 1965 and 1967 (Rosinski 1988).

By 1977, there were seventy-two such departments in medical schools across the country (Miller 1980). While this did not represent a substantial domination in ideology, the trend was not insignificant. However, this turn toward science to guide the shaping of the next generation of physicians was never inevitable: medical faculty were threatened by these calls for reform. Educationists were criticized for using alienating and harsh language and for demanding reforms that were unpalatable to the status quo (Miller 1980). A questionnaire of departments of medical education showed that funding and recognition were the biggest challenges educationists faced. Miller's history concluded in 1980 with a sense of frustration that his peers were reluctant to embrace methods for teaching and assessment driven by educational psychology research. Other scholars noted that changes in medicine had been made, but without apparent alteration to basic philosophies about how best to train the next generation of physicians. One called it a "history of reform without change" (Bloom 1988), although others acknowledged that some modifications did occur to attitudes and values among medical students (Kendall and Reader 1988).

And yet, by the end of the 1980s, medical education research would become firmly institutionalized in medical schools across the United States. Here, my history of medical education research meets the history I present in chapter 1. The 1970s and 1980s were a time of increased patient protest and patient consumerism, as exemplified by the Women's Health Movement. The financing of healthcare changed as managed care spread and corporatization ramped up. The emphasis on standardizing communication skills and developing more sensitivity toward patients, which teaching and learning the pelvic exam demonstrate, occurred more broadly for all types of clinical skills education. In this way, the development of the GTA program aligns with this larger history, which explains how and why it came to be institutionalized. While in chapter 1 I presented this process from the perspective of the GTA program, I now to look at ways that medical education researchers were able to coopt these programs and use them for their own professional interests. This had profound implications for how expertise and affect were reconfigured.

The Search for Objective, Reliable, and Valid Measures of Clinical Skills

As I claim throughout this book, the economic and political threats that the medical profession faced in the 1960s and 1970s created new articulation of power relations between physicians and patients—and between biomedicine and the public in general. In this new regime of affect, how was the profession to respond? A monopoly over knowledge production had shored up the profession's authority, but the professional dominance of medicine was waning. In chapter 1, I show how the Women's Health Movement successfully threatened the economic and cultural bases of the profession's authority over the pelvic exam. Thus, the profession needed to regain the public's trust in its members. It did so through medical education research's scientific production of knowledge about affect—about the capacities of physicians and patients to relate to one another.[9] Central to medical education research are best practices for teaching and learning about the physician-patient relationship. They turn the experience between a physician and patient into a discrete set of observable skills—and thus knowable, measurable, and calculable.

The 1960s and 1970, there was a rupture in consensus with regard to how a medical student could be judged and accredited as a physician. A shift occurred over the course of this time period in which assessment of knowledge was no longer sufficient unto itself. Led by medical education researchers, a movement began to assess the performance of medical students (Khan et al. 2013). This movement framed itself as a response to the increasingly dehumanizing practice of medicine due to growth in science and technology. The examples I provide in chapter 1 ("cows with fewer spigots") of how women were dehumanized in teaching the pelvic exam show this clearly. Editorials began to appear in medical journals about the lack of training about the basics of practicing medicine, such as the physical examination. According to physicians David Seegal and Arthur R. Wertheim, "One of the unexpected and disturbing results of the development of increasingly precise and useful diagnostic measures in the laboratory and x-ray departments is a significant and often alarming decrease in emphasis on the training of the medical student to perform with excellence the average comprehensive physical examination" (1962:476). Observing that trainees at the time were not overseen in performing a complete physical exam prior to graduating medical school, Seegal and Wertheim further argued, "If one grants that this procedure is often the core . . . in the physician's armamentarium, surely the medical school has the responsibility of arranging that each student's technique in this area by closely checked" (Seegal and Wertheim 1962:476). They further note some concern that trainees were failing their board exams due to their inability to perform the physical exam.[10]

The medical education journals of this period demonstrate on ongoing tension between the quest for objectivity via standardization—an "an ongoing preoccupation with the creation of more objective educational tools" (Rangel et al. 2016:28)—and skepticism about the feasibility or desirability of such a goal. For example, in a report on the 1970 Research in Medical Education conference, a summary of the proceedings noted that among the trends seen "was the need to establish criteria, especially those of performance, for medical students and practicing physicians. . . . It was pointed out that some medical schools are emphasizing the need for clinical, problem-solving skills more than the mastery of large amounts of content material" (Barnes et al. 1970:679). Assessing performance in order to assure that all licensed and practicing physicians were competent became a crucial issue for researchers in medical education. The tools for achieving this were increasingly to be found in science, particularly sciences of the social such as psychometrics. "In these texts, there is a pervasive assumption that legitimate knowledge in medical education is quantifiable. The significant uptake of psychometrics within medical education has been linked to this assumption, aiding the endeavour to improve objectivity, reliability and validity" (Rangel et al. 2016:28). The effect of this move can be seen as well in the quest for standardized criteria for evaluating medical students' performance of the pelvic exam.[11]

One important problem for the standardization of medical training was that educators were at the mercy of whoever happened to be present in the clinic at the time. Recall, for example, Charles's discussion of how the generation before him was trained to do pelvic exams: on women selected at random from the clinic. Here, the concerns of feminists about the exploitation of clinic patients aligned with those of medical education researchers. A stand-in was needed, a person who could be a model for medical students but who would not be exploited or dehumanized by the arrangement. A faculty member in a department of medical education in Scotland, Ronald M. Harden (Harden et al. 1975; Harden and Gleeson 1979) established the first objective structured clinical examination (OSCE) to address this issue. Harden developed the idea of having numerous stations where medical students would perform procedures and be evaluated on them. This involved medical educators selecting clinic patients specifically for the OSCE and then breaking up parts of the exam into smaller components for each student to complete in turn. Harden and colleague Gleeson argued that the ideal assessment should be valid, reliable, and practical.

> Is it valid? Does it measure what it is supposed to measure? Is there evidence for what the examiners think they have seen? Can the examiners generalize from what they have seen? . . . Is it reliable? Is the examination an objective assessment? Are the results accurate and consistent? Would other assessors agree with the examiner's interpretation of the student's behaviour? . . . Is it practical? Can the requirements for staff and accommodation be met? Can it cope with sufficient numbers of students? (Harden and Gleeson 1979:41)

Medical educators and sociologists of medical education will recognize the term OSCE. To foreshadow, the OSCE is now the preferred method for assessing clinical skills in trainees, but it uses simulated patients instead of actual patients. GTAs will often also do OSCEs alongside their regular teaching sessions to provide standardized evaluations of trainees' performance of the pelvic exam. The OSCE thus promised a scientific way to assure uniformity in training and objectivity in evaluation.

At the beginning of the 1980s, concerns about how to evaluate medical student performance ramped up. In particular, communication and interpersonal skills became key targets, and medical education researchers turned their attention to looking for techniques for managing affect while also furthering medicine's goal of standardization. As one physician-instructor argued in an article in the journal *Medical Education*, "Clinical medicine is above all else about communication between two people, it is about establishing an effective working relationship in which there is mutual trust" (Irwin, McClelland, and Love 1989:387).

Likewise, others noted the relationship between the style of practice of a physician and the desired outcome of the clinical encounter.

> Today's increased emphasis on the mind-body relationship . . . has brought about an exploration in medical school curricula of new ways to teach the affective skills needed by physicians. Studies have found that the mind-body relationship impacts on patient compliance with medical advice, on patient satisfaction with their physician, and on the data obtained by the physician from the patient. (Northup 1984:232)

Here, medical education researchers' concerns mirror the concerns of feminists, as I discuss in chapter 1. And yet, as the PTP critiques of co-optation predicted, the development of a relationship with the patient was more about "managing" the patient (compliance, satisfaction, information) than attending to the patient's lived experience. The politics of care become depoliticized as "affective skills."

In the process, the demarcation of objective, observable, and measurable skills for relating to patients was critical.

> What "communication skills" actually consist of has been specified concretely by behaviourally-oriented researchers . . . In particular, the empathetic verbal response, which acknowledges both the affect and the content of the other party's words, communicates attentiveness and respect. These in turn facilitate information gathering and the development of rapport. . . . Untrained students find it difficult both to elicit salient facts . . . and to cope with displays of patient emotion. (Winefield 1982:192)

These behaviorally oriented researchers (primarily psychologists—the heyday of sociologists in medical education had ended, though a few continued to work in medical schools) thus worked to turn the intersubjective experience of the physician-patient relationship into a measurable object anchored in concrete, observable actions that could be taught. In theory, all medical students could learn to communicate with empathy and respect. In this way, medical work in the clinical encounter was made inseparable from the emotional displays of physicians and their ability to "cope with" patients' emotions. For example, rapport is built with the patient through the proper choice of words and the way in which those words are spoken.

Those arguing for uniformity in teaching and learning these skills used evidence-based research in medical education to advance their position.

> It has become increasingly clear that how doctors communicate with patients affects the accuracy of their diagnoses, their patients' compliance, satisfaction and response to investigation and treatment. This has led many teachers of medical students to introduce training in these skills. Other teachers have remained sceptical [sic] about it even when faced with evidence from studies which have claimed that such training is effective. (Sanson-Fisher, Fairbairn, and Maguire 1981:33)

National governing bodies were listening. In the early 1980s, the Association of American Medical Colleges (AAMC) established a special panel to systematically review the education of physicians. This panel, the General Professional Education of Physicians and College Preparation for Medicine, for GPEP for short, was convened in 1981 and produced its final report, titled *Physicians for the Twenty-First Century*, in 1984. The Working Group on Fundamental Skills within GPEP "was particularly critical of the clinical education of medical students" (Nutter and Whitcomb 2001:3). It took aim at the lack of supervision for clinical clerkships, calling them "little more than unstructured apprenticeship experiences that contributed little to the overall learning objectives of the educational program" (Nutter and Whitcomb 2001:3). It recommended a more comprehensive review of clinical education for medical students. Accordingly, in 1985, the AAMC convened the National Invitational Conference on the Clinical Education of Medical Students, which sought to establish standards for medical student training and assessment. These national regulatory efforts set the stage for the kinds of experimentation that led to GTA programs, as medical schools were increasingly required to develop new modes of assessing performance on tasks like the pelvic exam.

Amid all of this debate and experimentation, medical education research was being entrenched firmly into the institutions of medicine. In 1987, the Society for Directors of Research in Medical Education was established, formalizing the informal work that physicians had been doing since the 1960s (Rosinski 1988). The number of specialty journals and grants increased, as did the number of advanced degree programs for teaching and learning in medicine. The Department of Medical Education at the University of Illinois at Chicago established a master's degree in Health Professions Education in the 1980s primarily for physicians seeking to gain expertise in teaching medical students— and conducting research on teaching and learning in medical school. The University of Southern California also established such a degree program, and other medical schools soon followed.[12]

Thus, throughout this period, the tools of science (objectivity, reliability, and validity), which had long been part of the medicine's quest for professional dominance emerged as a solution to another crisis of legitimacy, that of the uneven training of medical students. Medical education researchers were able to leverage this crisis to gain institutional support for their work by promising advances through the psy-sciences in governing the conduct of medical students and physicians. What is most fascinating about these debates is that they center the affective engagement between physician and patient as their object of attention. Accordingly, two intertwined technologies of affect emerged—the simulated patient and the communication and interpersonal skills checklist— both of which have shaped the way that many kinds of clinical sessions are practiced today.

The Simulated Patient and the Communication and Interpersonal Skills Checklist

In the effort to find objective, reliable, and valid measures of medical student performance through the deployment of research in medical education, researchers sought to include a new type of expert—the "nonphysician in medical education," as some literature would call them (Linn et al. 1986; Miller 1990; Stillman et al. 1990b; Stillman and Swanson 1987). The goal was to use trained laypeople to evaluate the performance of medical students on different types of clinical skills. Thus, two technologies emerged as solutions for standardizing these experiences: the communication and interpersonal skills checklist and the simulated patient.[13] With a standardized instrument—a checklist—medical education researchers believed that they could train and evaluate medical students' abilities to develop and manage the physician-patient relationship. The shift toward standardizing the pelvic exam that I discuss at the end of chapter 1 was part of this trend. As I show now, research on GTAs was central to the creation of these technologies in medical education research.

While simulation in the health professions has occurred since at least the sixteenth century (Buck 1991), the simulated patient arose in the 1970s through the work of medical education researchers. Physician Howard S. Barrows and neurology professor Stephen Abrahamson devised the "programmed patient" to address uniformity of training for neurology clerkship students. The function of a programmed patient "involves the simulation of disease by a normal person who is trained to assume and present, on examination, the history and neurological findings of an actual patient in the manner of an actual patient" (Barrows and Abrahamson 1964:803). Barrows and Abrahamson described how they trained an art model to portray an actual neurological case from their clinic and to fill out a questionnaire for each trainee to assess their performance. Barrows and Abrahamson concluded: "Not only does this technique avoid the problems incurred when an observer is present, it offers the far more important advantage of guaranteeing that the patient is constant for all students being tested" (Barrows and Abrahamson 1964:805). In this way, "programmed patients" offered the possibility of standardizing training and evaluation. Likewise, the "problems incurred" by the presence of a physician are similar to the concerns that led medical educators to develop GTA programs—namely, student anxiety and fear of making mistakes in front of senior physicians.

Physicians Ray Helfer and Joseph Hess likewise experimented with trained laypeople to assess trainees' skills, but their methods of evaluation were more rigorous and were derived from educational psychology. In the *Journal of Clinical Psychology*, they wrote:

> The ability of medical educators to assist students in developing the skills of interpersonal communication has been hampered by the inherent difficulty of making objective measurements of the actual performance of any given student or group of students. We often are dependent upon the subjective views of a single observer, or commonly no observer at all,

in our attempts to help medical students develop this skill. . . . Making objective measurements of interviewing skills not only enhances the probability of increasing the student's motivation but also provides an opportunity to construct research designs measuring the effectiveness of various instructional methods. (Helfer and Hess 1970:327)

Helfer and Hess recruited medical students' wives to play mothers of seriously ill children. These women were instructed in the details of their "child's" case and trained to use two objective instruments to assess the medical students' performance. The first was counting certain positive and negative behaviors and the second was a checklist of facts about the case (both medical and psychosocial) that the rater obtained. These tools were adapted from the interaction process analysis developed by social psychologist Robert F. Bales and educational psychologist Ned Flanders. It is interesting here that women were recruited to do this affective labor, a theme that I address further in chapters 3 and 4.

In 1974, at the University of Arizona, Paula Stillman began experimenting with trained actors, whom she called "patient instructors," to teach medical students and residents about medical interviewing in a standardized fashion using what came to be known as the Arizona Clinical Interview Rating Scale (Stillman et al. 1977). Observing interviews conducted by physicians "considered to be expert interviewers" (1977:1034),[14] Stillman and her colleagues (1977) defined sixteen skills that separated good interviewers from poor interviewers (grouped under the categories of organization, timeline, transitional statements, questioning skills, documentation, and rapport) and developed anchoring statements that described the behaviors to help raters assess performance on a one-to-five scale from poor to excellent. They also repeatedly tested the scale for reliability and validity using patient instructors, as well as an experienced physician and medical students, and concluded that "in addition to providing for outcome evaluation (e.g., grading decisions) the [scale] can furnish information useful for formative evaluation (e.g., monitoring of student progress to recommend further instruction) and can provide a valuable learning experience for the student" (Stillman et al. 1977:1037). In this way, Stillman introduced a seemingly objective method to capture the physician-patient relationship.

Research on GTA programs, which focused on their effectiveness for evaluating students' skills in a standardized way and quantifying their impacts on students, formed the backbone of work on formative assessment. One early study compared students' self-rating of their abilities to perform the exam successfully with GTAs' assessments and found only one key area of difference: technique (Johnson et al. 1975). Medical students were much more likely to believe they had not caused discomfort or pain to the "patient" than GTAs were.[15] In this way, the use of the GTA as a simulated patient demonstrates a new regime that valued affect. The fact that a medical student had hurt a patient *as determined by that patient* mattered for the official assessment of that student's performance. Gone was the era of referring her to a psychiatrist for being abnormal. Instead, a student would need more training. Thus, GTAs helped usher in an era in medical education research in which the embodied expertise of the patient—not just the expertise of the supervising physician—was significant in determining how competent a medical student was.

More studies in the 1980s used gold standard methods such as randomized control trials to compare students who had undergone traditional methods of teaching and learning the pelvic exam on manikins and clinic patients with those who went through GTA programs (Fang et al. 1984; Guenther, Laube, and Matthes 1983; Livingstone and Ostrow 1978; Nelson 1978; Plauché and Baugniet-Nebrija 1985; Shain, Crouch, and Weinberg 1982; Vontver et al. 1980). In one such study, physician Lewis H. Nelson divided medical students randomly into four groups who practiced on a manikin, a GTA, or both in different orders, and then compared their performance on another set of GTAs. Students who had practiced with GTAs demonstrated no significant difference in "professional manner, ability to recognize external anatomy, and understanding of the pelvic exam," but "appeared to be more gentle in their examination" (Nelson 1978:631). In addition, in students' self-rating of anxiety, those who had practiced only on a GTA *or* on a GTA and then a manikin, showed statistically significant reduction in their post-test measures compared to their pre-test. Here, then, was objective, scientific proof (following the rules of the medical education research game) that GTAs were effective at calming students down.

In a study published jointly in the *Journal of Medical Education*, physician Warren C. Plauché and GTA program coordinator Wendy

Baugniet-Nebrija (1985) developed more sophisticated measures. GTAs in their study completed a checklist ranking students' performance as "very good," "satisfactory," or "needs improvement" in several categories: "examination technique, professional demeanor, communication" skills, and method of patient education," which "were derived from the examination protocols" (Plauché and Baugniet-Nebrija 1985:872). Students used a five-point Likert scale (1 = strongly disagree to 5 = strongly agree) to rate measures such as "student comfort increased," "knowledge increased," "GTAs well prepared," and "learning experience successful." For all of these, 85 percent or more of students rated the experience a "5." According to GTAs, 27 percent of students had challenges communicating with the patient, such as "indiscreet language, speaking in a condescending way, talking 'over the patient's head' and failure properly to educate the patient" (Plauché and Baugniet-Nebrija 1985:874). Eighteen percent also caused discomfort due to "lack of gentleness, lack of concern or reassurance, and painful speculum or bimanual examinations" (Plauché and Baugniet-Nebrija 1985:874).

In all of these ways, a growing body of evidence coming out of medical education research verified that GTAs and other "programmed patients" or laypeople were effective in teaching clinical skills and ensuring that students were performing competently. GTAs in particular were scientifically vetted for their ability to improve student performance and reduce students' anxiety. Where laypeople, such as those who received pelvic exams, had such authority, the effect was twofold: on the one hand, it weakened the authority of physicians; on the other, it buttressed medical expertise by ensuring the competence of its providers (see chapter 3).

Toward the end of the 1980s, interest in other ways to use nonphysician educators expanded. In 1989, a clinical skills assessment alliance was formed in which medical education researchers played a key role in developing new best practices. "To resolve some of the continuing differences of opinion about the use of standardized patients within medical schools, it also seemed important to bring academic researchers into the field together with those faculty leaders who were most concerned about the practical problem of implementing such examinations" (Miller 1994:286). There was widespread evidence that simulation techniques were being increasingly used for both formative assessment—meaning used for training and teaching a set of behaviors or attitudes—and summative assessment—meaning, used for judging proficiency (Miller 1994). A survey that same year reported that nearly 70 percent of medical schools used simulated patients in some form. Teaching the breast and pelvic exam was the most popular use for simulated patients, but teaching interview skills and the entire or part of the physical exam was also popular (Stillman et al. 1990a). About half of the schools that used simulated patients had developed or adopted a checklist to guide the encounters.

These checklists became more sophisticated in focusing on more aspects of the physician-patient relationship associated with emotion. A checklist "involves an observer's rating a trainee's performance of several communication behaviors, using a numeric scale of ratings for low to high performance" (Duffy et al. 2004:498) and can thus capture emotion in quickly identifiable ways. One of the most commonly used communication and interpersonal skills checklists today was developed by Gregory Makoul, who holds a PhD in Communication Studies and has been internationally recognized for his expertise in physician-patient communication. The SEGUE Framework—which stands for "Set the stage, Elicit information, Give information, Understand the patient's perspective, and End the encounter"—consists of a list of observable tasks that are marked either "yes" for completed or "no" for not. These tasks include, for example, "make a personal connection during visit," "discuss how the health problem affects the patient's life," and "express caring, concern, and empathy" (Makoul 2001). Numeric assessments, such as Likert scales, likewise enabled patients or observers to rate things like how well a medical trainee put the patient at ease, how empathetic the trainee was, how confident and respectful, how nonjudgmental, and how well the trainee "maintained a comfortable and appropriate distance during the interview" (Cohen et al. 1996). I attend to the gendered, racialized, and economic ideologies that underpin these technologies in chapter 6.

All of this interest in simulated patients and the communication and interpersonal skills checklist altered not only medical school curricula but also licensing practices. In 1989, the Educational Commission for Foreign Medical Graduates (ECFMG) and the Liaison Committee on Medical Education (LCME) began developing tools for assessing clinical skills with simulated patients (Kassebaum and Eaglen 1999). In 1991, the LCME announced that all medical schools needed to implement some standardized method of assessing clinical skills. The AAMC backed up the LCME in 1992 with the report *Educating Medical Students*. That same year, the AAMC convened a Consensus Conference on the Use of Standardized Patients in the Teaching and Evaluation of Clinical Skills (Anderson 1993). This was also the year that the United States Medical Licensing Exam (USMLE) became a requirement, strengthening the power of the primary source of medical education research publications and funding, the National Board of Medical Examiners (NBME).

With this change, interest in and research of using simulated patients and checklists grew during the 1990s and continued into the early 2000s.[16] Thus, in 2002, at a meeting of twenty-seven experts on medical education research at the second Kalamazoo Consensus Conference on assessing communication skills, attendees agreed that "Professional conversation between patients and doctors shapes diagnosis, initiates therapy, and establishes a caring relationship. The degree to which these activities are successful depends, in large part, on the communication and interpersonal skills of the physician. . . . Valid, reliable, and practical measures can guide professional formation, determine readiness for independent practice, and deepen understanding of the communication itself" (Duffy et al. 2004:495).[17] Communication skills, the report states, "can be defined as specific tasks and observable behaviors," while interpersonal skills are "inherently relational" (Duffy et al. 2004:497). Interpersonal skills include:

> "(1) respect, including treating others as one would want to be treated; (2) paying attention to the patient with open verbal, nonverbal, and intuitive communication channels; (3) being personally present in the moment with the patient, mindful of the importance of the relationship; and (4) having a caring intent, not only to relieve suffering but also to be curious and interested in the patient's ideas, values, and concerns" (Duffy et al. 2004:498).

The report then details three methods for assessing these skills in medical trainees, including the use of checklists, patient satisfaction surveys, and written examinations. This consensus statement emphasizes throughout the importance of using science-driven, objective methods for assessing a medical trainee's performance on a set of skills that has been rigorously defined as a constellation of observable and measurable behaviors. The effect, thus, is to render the "inherently relational" experience that occurs between a physician and a patient into the same objectively knowable phenomenon as following disease-prevention techniques in surgery. In this way, the ability of medical education research to govern "at arms' length" through affect was strengthened.

In 2004, a further development in this process came in the form of the introduction to the USMLE of a component that focused exclusively on communication and interpersonal skills through the use of standardized patients. In order to be a licensed physician, every medical student thus had to pass a standardized exam of their ability to ask questions, convey empathy, and use the appropriate nonverbal communication skills. In this way, the use of the communication and interpersonal skills checklist and the use of simulated patients had fully merged with the main ways in which medical trainees' performance was assessed, including high-stakes licensing exams.

Thus, medical education research responded to the structural changes of the 1970s by standardizing how a medical trainee's ability to relate to patients would be assessed and taught. The key technologies at play were the checklist and simulated patient. Developing technologies such as checklists and simulated patients is also how medical education research, as a distinct form of expertise, has become central to reproducing the field of medicine through training the next generation of physicians. The technologies of the checklist and of simulation, both human and nonhuman, are constantly evolving and being improved upon as medical education research continues to proliferate. These technologies guide the GTA session today by providing the standardized materials (via the checklist) and the simulated patient (the GTA) for teaching the skills of the pelvic exam. Because GTA programs were incorporated into medical schools under this framework of standardization and simulation (rather than feminist models of care like the Pelvic Teaching Program analyzed in the previous chapter), they share much in common with other encounters medical students have with simulated patients. Such educational initiatives are jointly managed by the same knowledges and practices of clinical skills education, such as the proper verbal and nonverbal communication behaviors, as well as the correct emotional disposition of empathy toward the patient. These technologies of affect are produced through research by experts and serve to govern affect in medical education.

Too Relational? Affect as the Internal Limit of Medical Education Research

Medical education research today is a body of expertise that guides almost every area of teaching and learning in medical school, from premedical education at the bachelor's degree level to licensing at the graduate level. Departments of medical education have become a ubiquitous part of medical schools, where they address "increased public expectations relating to healthcare, societal trends towards increased accountability, educational developments, increased interest in what to teach and how to educate doctors and the need to train more doctors" (Davis, Karunathilake, and Harden 2005:665). According to the 2013 survey of member units by the Society for the Directors of Research in Medical Education, medical education research departments and offices receive considerable support from universities. The average budget for such units is around $1.3 million dollars, with about 88 percent of that coming as direct funds from the university.[18] Departments of medical education are typically made up of MD and PhD-level faculty members from a diversity of academic backgrounds, including psychology, communication, sociology, anthropology, history, literature, and philosophy.[19] These departments also include highly skilled and specialized staff who manage and oversee admissions programs, simulation centers, and grant research.[20] In this way, analyzing medical education research as a form of expertise allows me to consider how laypeople such as GTAs are able to wield authority and expertise in medical education, which I consider in chapter 3. Taken together, this network of knowledges and practices produces simulated patients and the communication and interpersonal skills checklist as technologies of affect.

The story that I tell in this chapter of the rise of simulated patients and the communication and interpersonal skills checklist from the meta-expertise of medical education research is one new mode of affective governance. I have posed the emergence of these technologies as curious objects that mix scientific expertise with the intersubjective experience of a clinical encounter. I am interested in what ruptures and exclusions occur in the shaping of such technologies as researchers of medical education grapple with the emotional lives and affective capacities of their subjects. If we can agree that it is not affect that is being standardized here, then what is the relationship between the seemingly objective science of medical education research and affect?

In *Parables for the Virtual*, Brian Massumi (2002) writes of a science, language, and measurability at the threshold of affect. In the chapter "Too-Blue," Massumi describes an experiment in which subjects were asked to match the color of a loved one's eyes recalled from memory to a selection of color samples. Subjects repeatedly chose colors that were too vibrant or exaggerated to actually exist as the color of someone's eyes. The friend's eyes are remembered as "too blue": "too saturated to match an object which is known to have a distinct hue" (Massumi 2002:210). The experimenter was attempting to standardize all the possible colors of eyes and experiences of those eyes into a limited set of options, whereas the subject of the experiment was remembering the experience of a loved one's eyes. Thus, the objective measure and the affect-saturated experience of the memory missed one another. The subject's experience was in excess of what the experimenter's standardized tool can capture.

In this way, the experiment got to a truth about the co-mingling of sociality, language, and affect. Language attempts to both standardize and convey the "ineffable singularity of experience" (Massumi 2002:211). A subject cannot remember a friend's eyes in this experiment because the affective *experience* of a loved one's eyes cannot fully be captured in language. In this way, the imposition of language produces a rupture in experience. Recall from the introduction that in Massumi's account (2002:213), affect is an experiential excess, a potentiality, that cannot be captured in the realm of the real (i.e., the empirical) without being transformed or translated in some way (i.e., an emotion is recognized affect; too-blue is the recognition of the color of an eye striking a subject).

This makes affect difficult for science to grapple with. As I show in this chapter and throughout the book, teaching and learning the pelvic exam has been difficult for medical educators because of its affective charge. However, the concepts of objectivity and empiricism provide a lens for understanding the relationship between science and affect.

Affect forms a boundary that science cannot and should not cross over into: specifically, the realm of potentiality in which affect resides is the "limit of objectivity which sciences approach from within their own operation" (Massumi 2002:229). To cross over into the realm of affect is to lose all claims on objectivity. To experience empathy with a patient in the pelvic exam, for example, is to step beyond the medical profession's historical obsession with scientific ways of knowing. In this way, the objects produced by science must be treated discretely and with repeatable effects. Empathy in the pelvic exam has to become an object that a GTA can mark "Well Done" or "Needs Improvement" in a regular fashion across all students. This turning of affect into something objective occurs through processes of translation, in which "discursive and institutional practices manage a certain regularity and predictability" (Massumi 2002:218) as the object moves through different spaces. As affect passes out of the pure experience, it must be translated in order to be recognizable and understood by the knowledge and practices of science. Empathy in the pelvic exam thus becomes an object that can be measured in the same way by different GTAs teaching different medical students across different medical schools and clinical contexts. It becomes a thing that can be grasped and known by expert practices.

I argue that the communication and interpersonal skills checklist and the simulated patient (such as the GTA) are technologies of affect. Medical education research—because it is a science—cannot and should not traffic in affect; the "ineffable singularity of experience" (Massumi 2002:211) in which affect resides is the limit of this kind of research. The physician-patient relationship is "too relational" by virtue of being an experience, just as the color of a loved one's eyes is 'too blue' (or too brown or whatever you experience). As such, to make the relationship intelligible to the technologies of objectivity and standardization that medical education research values, it must be rendered regular and predictable as it moves around clinical and social spaces. Affect must be brought up to the level of language in order to be discursively captured with the tools of contemporary medical education research. This is what I mean by the checklist being a technology of affect. It captures in simple language and observable behaviors the elements of experience between physician and patient. It manages affect, it attempts to capture affect, and yet affect always escapes such attempts at signification. As such, affect is unruly and always already a threat to such technologies. Medical students who excel at performing to the checklist may find themselves completely lost in the clinical encounter. Dealing with patients' strong emotions—grief or especially anger—can derail the most accomplished physician. A patient's affectively too-sticky body may evoke emotions in the best-trained physician. Or, in the reverse, a physician whose body is surfaced by affects such as disgust and exclusion due to historical legacies of oppression may struggle to contain the clinical encounter into the checklist.[21]

In this way, I find the concept of technologies of affect useful for capturing the tension between the drive toward objectivity and standardization in medical education research and the lived experienced of the physician-patient relationship. It accounts for emotions and bodies and for the intended and unintended ways that our capacities to act and be acted upon by one another produce both regularities and ruptures in the standard way that the encounter ought to be conducted. Given the centrality of expertise in these technologies, what is the nature of the kind of labor that those people in whose bodies affective forms of authority are lodged perform in medical education? I turn to this question in the next chapter.

3

"This Power with My Body"

Intimate Authority in GTA Sessions

Grace was almost finished training to become a gynecological teaching associate when she had a momentary pause. Up until that point, she had felt completely comfortable with the work. She had a background in sexual health and had been working as a standardized patient when a coworker told her about GTA work. "I thought, oh, that sounds interesting!" she said. I probed: what made the work interesting?

> [It] made me feel good about myself . . . I felt like I was really making a difference and I was using my body to do that. Strange as that may seem . . . I've always been self-conscious about my body. . . . [but] . . . when my son was born, I remember feeling like my body had purpose. I have breasts that have purpose that is not sexual. And I felt the same way about doing this job. . . . I have this power with my body and it's not sexual.

Thinking about her motivation to start training, she said, "I got involved because I really thought I could make a difference." She wanted to improve the provision of reproductive healthcare and also provide a better educational experience for medical students. That the pay was good and the schedule flexible was also very appealing.

Training went smoothly until she herself had to perform the exam on her training partner's body.

> I was a little concerned. . . . I got really comfortable with that person, and then it dawned on me one day, you know, you're going to have to do this for somebody other than just this one person that you've really bonded with. And, oh, by the way, you might have a male student. And then I started thinking, I can't believe I'm getting ready to do this.

Grace was specifically worried about working with men as her students.

> Part of the training, before I had my first official student, I had a mock session . . . with two males. And it was like, you know, facing my fears head on immediately. And they were great. I mean, it couldn't have gone any better. . . . That just really paved the way for me to be comfortable. . . . [After that] I really did not have any reservations about doing it.

For Grace, there was a duality about the intimacy of this kind of work that both drew her to it and gave her pause. On one hand, the act of using her body to improve reproductive healthcare in such an intimate fashion gave her a sense of purpose and power in her embodiment. And on the other hand, the notion of doing such an intimate form of work with strangers—especially men—seemed for a moment like it might be too strange. Ultimately, Grace realized that even in such intimate forms of work, she could command authority and that this job could fit both her financial needs and her commitments to reproductive healthcare.

Many of the GTAs whom I interviewed spoke in one way or another about this duality, about the unusual co-mingling of intimacy and authority that animate their work. Marie said: "It's an intimate and it's also, in many ways, a sacred moment, to share the body. . . . It's very . . . empowering to be able to share my body like that and be respected and teach people who are fascinated by it." GTAs spoke in various ways of this intimacy, whether or not they made the connection to feminism explicit. They also spoke of it in describing their relationships with their coworkers. There are very few other jobs in which one learns hands-on how the position of a coworker's cervix changes over the course of their menstrual cycle.

GTA work puts together two seemingly contradictory realms: intimacy and paid labor. In this chapter, I unpack these tensions, contradictions, and co-minglings. I argue that the intimate labor that GTAs do relies upon care and attentiveness to their bodies, their coworkers' bodies, and the bodies and emotions of their students. They stand in for actual patients in this way, providing their bodies for medical students to practice on, even as they work as para-professionals in medical education by providing feedback and assessment. The contradictions inherent in their work are captured by an older term for their role: "patient instructor." Their work relies on both the intimacy and vulnerability that comes with being a patient *and* the authority that being an instructor in a medical school confers. This analysis aligns with my goal in this book of examining affective governance in medical education by turning my attention to the workers who labor in intimate ways to prepare medical students to embody the new values and techniques of the physician-patient relationship. To this analysis I bring yet another layer of intimacy: that of you and me, reader. I did this work myself for over a decade, and in this chapter, I draw on my own intimate knowledge to inform my empirical analysis. I become in this chapter, perhaps, an immodest witness to my subject matter.[1]

"Nonphysician Experts" and Intimate Labor in Medical Education

The widespread growth of nonphysician experts in medical education has opened up the educational space to new forms of expertise and new types of workers. Simulated patients are a subset of this group, of which GTAs are an even more specialized subset. In this chapter, I argue that GTAs perform intimate labor, using haptic knowledge of their bodily interiors and deploying deep forms of attentiveness to their bodies, their coworkers' bodies, and their students' bodies and emotions, in order to produce more caring physicians and more patient-friendly pelvic exams.[2] I follow feminist scholars Eileen Boris and Rhacel Salazar Parreñas in theorizing the work of GTAs as paid labor that "promote[s] the physical, intellectual, affective, and other emotional needs of strangers, friends, family, sex partners, children and elderly, ill, or disabled people" (2010:2). Such intimate labor involves "bodily and psychic intimacy" (Boris and Parreñas 2010:2), and it often overlaps with reproductive or affective labor, in that it is about fostering new members of a workforce through close bodily and emotional interactions. Attentiveness is a key aspect of intimate labor—attentiveness to one's own body and to the bodies and emotions of others.[3]

As sociologist Viviana Zelizer argues, what makes for *intimacy* in intimate forms of labor is that these relations "depend on particularized knowledge received, and attention provided by, at least one person—knowledge and attention that are not widely available to third parties" (2005:14). Furthermore, "The knowledge involved includes such elements as shared secrets, interpersonal rituals, bodily information, awareness of personal vulnerability, and shared memory of embarrassing situations" (Zelizer 2005:14). I draw from this definition to characterize the work of GTAs as intimate. It involves the exchange—for money—of deeply felt knowledge about the interiors of one's body, to which medical students would otherwise have no access as even regular clinic patients do not have this repertoire of knowledge. Furthermore, the work GTAs perform is intimate in that it exposes them to the "personal vulnerability" of medical students. As I discussed in chapter 1, GTA programs originated and have become popular in part because of medical students' anxiety about doing pelvic exams. Part of this anxiety is the fear of embarrassing themselves and appearing incompetent in front of their peers and their supervisions. In this way, GTAs' intimate labor involves exchanges of trust. GTAs "willingly share such knowledge and attention in the face of risky situations" (Zelizer 2005:15), whereas medical students give GTAs access to knowledge about their vulnerabilities. According to Zelizer, intimate labor always involves relations of caring, which she defines as involving both "sustained attention" and efforts to "enhance the welfare" of the person for whom care is being provided (2005:17).

What makes the work of GTAs *labor* is that it produces value. Specifically, it is a form of reproductive labor, in that it "involves embodied and affective interactions in the service of social reproduction" (Boris and Parreñas 2010:7). Economist Isabella Bakker (2007) argues that education and training in the workforce are forms of reproductive labor, since they create new workers, and Zelizer likewise agrees that educational labor produces "human capital" (2010:269). In this way, the educational mission of the GTA session is a form of labor that seeks to produce and shape trainees who embody the values of the medical profession. GTAs establish and build relationships—between one another, between themselves and their students, and between their students and those students' future patients. The goal of this labor is to craft more patient-friendly, sensitive, and comfortable physicians. In this way, the labor that GTAs perform is affective, in that it produces new forms of sociality and community among medical trainees.[4]

GTA Programs Today: Para-Professionalism and Precarity

I studied GTA programs at three major medical schools in Chicago, which share many of the same characteristics. However, because there are so few GTAs relative to the number of medical students and faculty in Chicago, I interviewed GTAs across the country. GTA programs nationally emphasize similar manual and communication skills.[5] As I show in this section, the intimate labor that GTAs perform sits at the intersections of para-professionalism and precarity. GTAs use their bodily knowledge to stake claims on authority in medical education, but their work is characterized by instability and lack of institutional grounding. In this way, their intimate labor is "situated in the labor market—both formal and informal—and subject to market forces and ideological views on gender, ethnicity, race, and sexuality, and structural constraints" (Boris and Parreñas 2010:9).

In a typical session, a GTA walks two to three medical students through a complete breast and pelvic exam. This usually lasts around an hour and a half. GTAs teach both communication skills and manual-technical skills, guided by the checklist I described in chapter 2. The two biggest variations in how GTA sessions are run is whether the breast exam is taught and whether the GTA teaches alone. In Chicago, GTAs tend to "team-teach," or teach in pairs, so that one GTA takes the role of instructor while the other GTA takes the role of the patient. At a few programs in Chicago and more nationwide, GTAs embody both roles simultaneously. The GTA on the table (in patient role) is always encouraged to give feedback or speak up if the student causes pain or discomfort and in most cases, will exclusively teach any internal exam. The GTAs with whom I spoke expressed different preferences for being instructor or patient or teaching solo or in pairs, depending on their teaching style, level of experience, and their relationships with the other GTAs. Team-teaching, as can be imagined, requires a great deal of intimacy with coworkers. On the other hand, it offers some protection, as it allows the partner of the GTA in the patient role to watch over the students from the other side of the table.

GTAs teach a set of communication skills that have become more or less standard across all formal clinical skills education. First, GTAs focus on teaching the medical students to use neutral, clinical language.

Medical jargon is to be avoided, but so, too, are colloquialisms that could be misconstrued as sexual. Words such as "touch" or "feel" are replaced with the words "inspect," "check," or "examine," collectively referred to by the acronym "ICE." Words such as "put" or "stick" are replaced with the more neutral "insert." For example, a medical student would be taught to use the phrase "I'm going to examine you now" instead of the "I'm going to feel you now," or "I will insert a finger" instead of "I'm going to stick a finger in you." Second, GTAs focus on how to walk the patient through the exam using "talk before touch." This communication skill involves informing the patient at every step of the way what is about to happen and what its purpose is. For the pelvic exam, the most important of these skills is the "neutral touch," whereby medical students learn to place the back of their hand on the inside of the patient's thigh, usually near the knee, and provide a verbal warning ("I'm going to begin") before making contact with the genitals.

Following American College of Obstetricians and Gynecologists (ACOG) clinical guidelines, a complete pelvic exam consists of three parts. The first tends to be an examination of the external genitalia and anal region. The medical student learns such techniques as checking the lymph nodes, pubic hair, and labial folds for signs of sexually transmitted infections (STIs) or cancer. In some programs, medical students also learn to check the anal region for hemorrhoids or STIs, and/or to check two sets of glands just inside the vagina. The second part of the pelvic exam is the speculum exam. Medical students often learn techniques to help relax the patient and cue the patient into the use and purpose of the speculum. Different techniques are used depending on the type of speculum, as metal and plastic specula work differently, but in general, GTAs teach medical students to move the speculum down and away from the anterior structures of the vagina (such as the urethra, which can be scraped or pinched). GTAs also typically teach students to insert the speculum on a slight oblique angle, again to avoid the anterior structures. Finally, GTAs teach medical students how to remove the speculum without allowing it to pinch the cervix or slide out fully open. The third part of the pelvic exam is the bimanual exam. This involves inserting one or two fingers into the vagina and placing the other hand on the patient's lower abdomen in order to use both hands to jointly palpate the internal structures. Medical students learn to locate the cervix, manipulate it to assess for pain, test its firmness and smoothness for signs of cancer or pregnancy, and then check the size and position of the uterus. In some programs, the medical students also learn to do a rectal exam to check for rectal polyps and examine the rectovaginal septum.

Most GTAs said that training occurred on the job and over a long period of time. Many began with a one- or two-day workshop in which they are exposed to all of the same materials as medical students regarding the pelvic exam, including articles, chapters from anatomy books, and lecture slides. Then, typically, they practiced the exam on one another, getting the experience both of walking someone through the exam on their own body *and* knowing what it feels like to actually do the exam on another person (which I discuss in chapter 5). Then, GTAs either observe their coworkers or stay in the patient role on the table for months, sometimes as long as a year, until they feel comfortable taking on the role of instructor. During this time, GTAs learn "the script,"[6] which is a more or less standardized way of teaching the exam, based on the checklist that they use afterward to evaluate students. At one program in Chicago, the script is literally a written document, which details word for word what should be said to medical students and is given to new GTAs to memorize. Once GTAs have done so, the coordinator or a senior GTA observes them teaching a group of medical students in order to certify them as fully independent instructors. I say "certify," but there are no formal certificates, nor are there any annual performance evaluations. The length of their experience on the job and the lack of any complaints from students or coworkers justify their continued employment.

The level of specialization and detailed knowledge that GTAs possess stands in contrast to the contingent nature of their employment. The contingent nature of their work tracks alongside national trends toward precarity in higher education—decreasing numbers of salaried positions and increasing amounts of contract-based work—the effects of which are deeply gendered (Zheng 2018). These labor conditions are tied to the concerns that early feminist GTAs had, which I discuss in chapter 1, and which led them to consider striking. GTA work tends to be seasonal and sessions are held in the evenings or on weekends—prime hours for caregivers, thus limiting the pool of who can do this work. GTAs in Chicago tend to be paid per event, while other GTAs may be paid hourly. The average pay nationally is about $55 per hour, while in Chicago a typical "event" is paid $175–$220 in total. In Chicago, in order to maximize travel time (since GTAs work all over the city and its suburbs), an event involves two sessions, so a GTA can expect to work with six students per night. On a longer day such as a weekend, a GTA may do four sessions total, with on average twelve students altogether. During "pelvic exam" season, a GTA may work two weeknights and one weekend day each week. This means that a GTA may potentially receive twenty-four pelvic exams in one week, though precautions are in place to make sure this doesn't happen without additional compensation.[7]

GTAs most frequently work through coordinators, who handle the scheduling and liaise between the GTAs and the medical schools. Coordinators handle any conflicts that may arise, though such conflicts are rare. Coordinators and GTAs tend to be paid as independent contractors, which means that they are not officially employees of the medical school and must file taxes accordingly. This also means that they receive no benefits from the schools they work for, such as retirement or health insurance (again, signaling the parallels of this work with other growing forms of precarity in the university).[8] While the GTAs with whom I spoke did not rely on this work for their primary income, some of them were able to work full-time as simulated patients. Most of them had full-time jobs and used GTA work to supplement that income. This was very much the case for me: I started working as a GTA while in college, continued in order to supplement my meager income in my first job, and found it a very helpful financial resource while living on a graduate stipend in the increasingly expensive city of Chicago.

GTA sessions tend to take place in medical school simulation centers or, more rarely, in outpatient clinics after hours. These rooms tend to be set up like regular exam rooms, with an exam table (including stirrups) and other supplies available.[9] The medical school provides all of the supplies to the GTA: specula, lubrication, gloves, and so forth. Some GTAs bring hand-mirrors or cloth hospital gowns of their own. While I was working as a GTA, we liked to joke about our "work uniform" being a favorite pair of socks we'd bring to keep our feet warm. Some GTAs purchase their own lubrication, since multiple exams with the low-quality lubrication provided by medical schools can cause problems.

While my focus in this book is on medical education, GTAs teach a variety of health professions students, including physicians' assistants, nursing students (undergraduate level and advanced practice level), chiropractors, and others. GTAs will sometimes also teach foreign-educated medical residents and sexual assault nurse examiners, though these sessions look different. There are also occasions when a GTA will not teach but only serve as a model for the purposes of evaluating a student's performance (such as during an objective structured clinical examination, discussed in chapter 2).

"Patient Instructors": Intimate Authority in the GTA Session

If intimate labor involves "particularized knowledge received, and attention provided by" a worker and this knowledge and attention are not "widely available to third parties" (Zelizer 2005:14), then GTA work is in many ways exemplary. The extensive training that GTAs undergo means that they develop a highly detailed stock of bodily knowledge about how the pelvic exam feels when performed on them. As I outlined in chapter 1, this knowledge is what makes them valuable to medical education, and in the context of intimate labor, it is how they *produce* value by using it to train medical students. Their authority, then, is intimate: it is based on deeply felt—to the point of being visceral—knowledge of their bodies that I call "haptic knowledge."

Sylvia, a GTA with ten years of experience, said, "It's knowledge gained from experience, gained from experience of having [*laughs*] having lots and lots and lots of exams." Sylvia's laughter in the middle of the sentence animates her emphasis on just how many exams she had to have in order to know her body that well. Similarly, Beth is a GTA who had been teaching in the same program for eight years at the time of our interview. "At some point when [she] did the math," she determined she had received "at least more than a thousand pelvics in [her] life."[10] She elaborated:

> But as far as people who can give accurate feedback on, is that my ovary, how far do you need to move your fingers this way or that way to be able to palpate my uterus, things like that. I am absolutely an expert on how to do this exam on my body. . . . I just have a huge amount of practice at it.

Nearly all GTAs with whom I spoke said that they can tell simply from feel whether students are doing the technique correctly or inserting the speculum appropriately. Their haptic knowledge comes from "lots and lots and lots" of experience that is acquired slowly and layered into the body. This knowledge is uniquely haptic: it is about the sensorial experience of pressure on her body's interiority. It resides deep in the viscera of the body and in a repertoire of interior feelings that most patients will never develop.

While the term "patient instructor" isn't as widely used anymore and stands among a myriad of terms for essentially the same type of job, I like what this term says about the nature of GTAs' work. GTAs use their haptic knowledge to stake claims of authority in the teaching encounter, when their roles as stand-ins for patients might otherwise render them subordinate. For example, Beth said:

> I'm the one in there with the knowledge. And it's the knowledge that puts you in control. . . . It doesn't matter if I'm wearing a paper gown and, you know, lying there in lithotomy position [in a reclined position with feet in the stirrups]. I am so clearly the one running the show. I am the one who is imparting my information to them, giving them the instructions on what they need to do, and, you know, providing answers to their questions and coaching. . . . There's really never any doubt in my mind then that I'm in control in that room.

Beth's unique claims to knowledge allow her to transcend typical practices that emphasize passivity and docility of the patient in the pelvic exam. The paper gown, the positioning of her body, all of this is second to her claims of authority; "instructor" takes precedence over the ways patients are typically positioned in the clinical encounter. GTAs' intimate labor thus relies on vulnerable and close bodily contact with strangers, and yet does not track along the same dynamics that scholars of body labor have identified (Gimlin 2007; Kang 2003, 2010; Underman 2011; Wolkowitz 2006). Their work is of course structured by the institutional context within which they labor. Because the knowledges and practices of medical education research have widened to include them, today's GTAs have tenuous legitimacy in medical education.

Samantha highlighted the importance of the instructor side of the patient instructor duality as she described the challenges of bringing GTA programs into new educational spaces:

> [Sometimes] I think there is a perception that we can be a person for the students to practice [on]. . . . The [medical school] will teach the students the exam and then you need somebody that is willing to have the exam performed on them and it is terrific if they have all the right parts and it's great if they kind of know where those parts are. . . . But not necessarily . . . realizing the depth of knowledge and training . . . having the skills to teach that exam . . . it's not just . . . knowing where your cervix is but being able to sensitively, comfortably, knowledgably teach that workshop. . . . And not everybody can do that. Some people could be a model but not effectively teach the workshop.

In other words, the emphasis falls on "being respected for being knowledgeable but also being a good teacher," as Samantha explained. GTAs are not just models for the exam. They use their haptic knowledge to teach medical students the pelvic exam, but they also use their knowledge, skills, and training about *teaching* to stake claims of authority. In this way, GTAs' authority as "patient instructors" sits at complex interstices between embodiment and science. It is this strange seemingly contradictory set of knowledges that I seek to capture with my term "intimate authority," which describes how in this form of work, intimacy and authority are in fact not opposed but co-productive.

However, because of the broader institutional structure within which they work, there are limits to GTAs' intimate authority. In the occupational hierarchy of the clinic, physicians have historically been at the top and maintain this position despite calls for interprofessional collaboration (Crawford, Omery, and Seago 2012; Matziou et al. 2014). While networks of expertise have been extended through nonphysicians, a story I tell in chapter 2, in the actual work of educating trainees, physicians' position of authority in medical education has been difficult to unseat. Even obliquely, the specter of the physician is always in the background of the session, throwing doubt on GTAs' authority. For example, Emory said:

When [you] have . . . a physician in the room with you, you can sort of get that extra level of medical knowledge there which you might miss with the GTA, who is very knowledgeable, although not necessarily trained in the medical field. . . . I guess there is a tradeoff there between having the physician expertise in the room with you, adding other tidbits of knowledge, versus having the patient who can [answer] to a better extent how this exam is personally affecting them.

In this way, the intimate authority of the GTA was certainly respected and valued by the medical students, but it stood in sharp contrast to the "extra level" of medical knowledge possessed by physicians. In this way, the intimate authority of GTAs is bound in time and place, as well as by social and cultural practices. As Boris and Parreñas argue: "Regardless of temporality, these labors all rely on the maintenance of precise social relations between employers and employees or customers and providers" (2010:3). The maintenance of the knowledge/authority hierarchy is one such social relation. Program coordinator Donna made the maintenance of authority an issue of "hands" and "communication":

[The GTA session is] less anxiety-provoking [for medical students] than if . . . there was a medical doctor in the room. . . . For the students, it's very constructive, it's very supportive. I think they feel like they're working in a partnership with the patient instructor. . . . They can ask questions and not feel like they should know this . . . [but the GTAs] can't answer questions about, you know, well, what if I found this, what if I feel that, you know? They can't do that. They can only teach . . . what the students should be doing with their hands and what they should be doing with their communication.

This distinction in types of knowledge (what to do with their hands and communication versus questions about pathology) highlights the point I make throughout this book about the role of the GTA program: this is an encounter about *affect*, and thus, the expertise that matters is how the patient (the GTA) *feels*. GTAs' work is to teach "hands" and "communication," but it is also equally about *taking care of* the medical students: reducing their anxiety, supporting them, not making them feel incompetent. In this way, their intimate labor is shaped by the context of their work. Their authority is valued by the institution of medical education, but it is specific and cordoned off.

Becoming a GTA: Caring Commitments and Entanglements of Money and Love

The commodification of care under capitalism means that new forms of paid labor have emerged in which intimacy—such as bodily closeness and attentiveness—is both the mode of work and the product that is exchanged for money (Boris and Parreñas 2010; Ducey 2010; Weeks 2007). GTA work is exemplary in this way. GTAs are almost always motivated by some form of caring commitment, be it to students or patients, to do this very intimate form of labor; at the same time, the flexibility of the work and the amount of money that can be made doing it are attractive as well. As in other forms of intimate labor, acts of love and work for money are interconnected (Boris and Parreñas 2010).

These complicated entanglements of money and love start even before GTAs begin training. The coordinators I spoke to said that they tend to recruit through personal networks rather than through formal advertisements. This ensures that interested applicants understand the nature of the work and are doing it for the "right" reasons, such as having a commitment to education. When I probed about what a "wrong" reason might be, I was given both an explicit and practical answer about not being in it just for the money and a more ill-defined and implicit response about screening out those who might be motivated for sexually exhibitionist reasons.[11] In this way, from the beginning, GTAs' work blends economic concerns with politics of care. The result of such recruitment strategies, however, is that GTA networks in various cities tend to be more or less internally homogenous. Almost all of the GTAs in my sample were college-educated and white, although there were exceptions. Most—but not all—were women. While GTAs need to have an intact uterus and cervix to do this work, there is no requirement that they present normatively as women.[12] A few identified as genderqueer at the time of our interviews. In addition, several transitioned after quitting, although I did not interview any men who were living as such while working as GTAs. Given that "embodied identities based on gender, race, nation, and class shape the meaning of intimate labor" (Boris and Parreñas 2010:11), I suspect that the largely white, middle-class, and educated composition of the GTA workforce lends to its authority in medical contexts. And yet, because these are predominantly women, the work is structured by gendered expectations of who a good teacher is (a topic I take up in chapter 4).

Care, as I discussed in chapter 1, is an affective engagement, a material investment in the world and the wellbeing of another person or object. In this way, GTAs care for patients, and before them medical students, through their intimate labor. The dominant reason that GTAs gave for doing this work was that they wanted to improve medical students' education and/or improve reproductive healthcare. Yet most also cited the pay and the flexibility of work schedules. This type of work, like all work in our current historical moment, sits at complex interstices of contingency and flexibility under capitalism (Weeks 2011). As Anna worded it, "I am very glad that it is well-compensated. I do ask myself sometimes, would you still do this if it were not well-compensated or as a volunteer? And my answer is, I might still do it, you know, like a couple times a year as a volunteer." Marie provided an exemplary response about the relationship between pay and "dedication" to improving the exam experience for patients:

> It's not just for the money because . . . it's mostly part-time and supplemental pay. So . . . there's something to be said for people's dedication. . . . As a patient . . . I know how uncomfortable some of these exams can be, and how they've been for me, and . . . I want to improve the quality of that experience and improve that respect for women.

These politics of care were sometimes explicitly named as a feminist politics of care or were identified as explicitly political in other ways. For example, Marie described her initial attraction to the work as "a very feminist thing to do . . . to . . . teach people how to basically respect women and how to have a sensitive and respectful and professional interaction with them." Beth described her involvement in various feminist causes and saw her work as a GTA as going hand in hand with her other activism. She explained: "I'm very, very political about medical care and about what I think is really wrong in it and what I think is good and, you know, what I think needs to change."

However, in other ways, GTAs' paid labor is intimately connected to their care for others, even if they do not name it outright as political. For example, Ingrid spoke of her motivation to work as a GTA as coming from her preexisting commitment to sexual assault survivors.

[If sexual assault survivors] could have a better gynecological exam . . . then I felt like I was contributing. . . . It was also sort of an empowering idea that you could be using your own body in such a positive way. . . . This is how to create a comfortable woman-positive environment. This is how to encourage more female patients to really know their own anatomy and to take an active role in their healthcare. [Historically], you lay almost flat on the table. You don't see anything that's going on. All of this stuff is just being done to you. Nothing is explained. And it's kind of insulting and infantilizing. And it's also stressful for women to have to go through that. So, I feel like we're teaching [students] more than just a technique. We're also teaching them a way of thinking of their female patients. And I think that's something that can carry through to the other things that are important to me.

Ingrid's response was fairly typical of all the GTAs I spoke with. She anticipates the future benefits of what she does, layering this anticipation on a construction of the past (and current) state of healthcare. In this way, GTA work involves modes of caring and attentiveness to commitments for all patients who receive pelvic exams as part of routine medical care. That Ingrid mentions the importance of teaching "a way of thinking of their female patients" underscores as well forms of affective labor that involve shaping relationships between medical students and their future patients. Ingrid seeks to develop medical students' affective capacities of care, respect, and sensitivity.

Gretchen also gave an answer that emphasizes the multiple ways GTA work evokes various entanglements of relationality:

Every time I say this is my job, I hear somebody's terrible pelvic exam story. . . . So this is my way of making these easier for other women directly, and also kind of troubling the way that we do medical education so that the patient has more authority. . . . To like teach [students] about women's bodies, but also to teach them how to do some empowerment with women. Yeah. I totally love it. That's absolutely my purpose.

In this way, GTA work constantly traffics in multiple forms of interconnectedness and relationality. Gretchen is connected to her fellow pelvic exam patients through the intimate sharing of "terrible pelvic exam stories." Her labor also seeks to connect physicians and patients, to challenge historical relations that neglect care in order to rearticulate the importance of the patient's personhood. Thus, the labor that GTAs perform is about more than the skills of the exam: it is about producing affective ties between physicians and patients. In this way, GTAs do exchange intimate forms of labor on their own bodies for money, but their work also involves the production of care and the formation of social relations between physicians and patients that are shaped by respect.

It is interesting to contrast GTAs' accounts of their motivations with the evolution of the GTA program as it was coopted by medical education and with some of the accounts I heard from program coordinators and medical educators. GTAs almost always explicitly mentioned care for hypothetical or actual other patients as their motivation, and yet the program as a whole has evolved to be about caring for medical students. As I outline in the next chapter, GTAs deploy their intimate authority and their close attention in order to provide students with a low-risk space in which to experience their first pelvic exam. In this way, while GTAs may individually and directly be motivated by care for patients, the institutional and structural position of the program within medical education redirects their caring energies. Their motivation is to care for patients, but their work is to care for medical students— reducing their anxiety and helping them develop the appropriate affects and habits now valued by medical education. This way, GTAs' work is about producing medical students as certain kinds of subjects under new regimes of affective governance: confident but caring, versed in science but skilled at managing relationships with other staff and especially with patients.

Sharing Bodies of Intimate Knowledge

Intimacy denotes vulnerability, but also pleasure (Zelizer 2005). The work GTAs do may be precarious and flexible, and it may involve intense bodily contact with strangers, but GTAs take pleasure in the intimacies of the work. My interviews revealed joy taken in sharing hidden knowledge about their bodies, as well as unique camaraderie with their coworkers. And, as an interviewer and myself a former GTA, I found some of my most pleasurable moments in conversations about the joys of sharing intimate knowledges. What these data demonstrate is that, for GTAs, the pleasure of intimacy is both necessary for doing their jobs and part of the *work* involved.

GTAs spoke in various ways about the moments when medical students located parts of their (the GTAs') anatomy. These moments when medical students connected both with the anatomical knowledge that they were acquiring and with the intimate interiors of the GTAs' bodies seemed almost to exist beyond language. For example, Ingrid explained:

> No matter how tired I am when I go to do one of these sessions . . . the first time a student actually feels, during a bimanual exam, oh my god, that is a uterus, or, you know, they're using a speculum for the first time and, oh my god, that's what a cervix looks like, or they feel an ovary . . . it sounds kind of hokey, but the . . . the kind of intensity of the . . . experience is very gratifying . . . even when it's not a very comfortable exam and I have to do a lot of adjustment in working with the student. . . . I was their first pelvic. They're never going to have to do another first pelvic. . . . I take sort of pride in that.

There is thus something unspeakably pleasurable about sharing this kind of intimacy with medical students. Ingrid speaks of "the intensity of the experience" that she takes pride in. She connects with the excitement students experience when they feel her anatomy for the first time— when they feel this kind of anatomy, usually so hidden and private, for the first time. Likewise, Gretchen described her favorite kind of student:

> I really like students who are curious. Who are excited [*laughs*]. . . . I get so jazzed when somebody like opens the speculum and my cervix pops

up and they're real into it. Oh, look, it's the cervix! They're my favorite. So no matter how inexperienced or ham-handed they are, it's fine, just as long as they have that sort of spirit of curiosity about it.

Ingrid, Gretchen, and the other GTAs with whom I spoke take pleasure in these experiences of sharing intimate knowledge with students. They find pleasure and pride in such attentiveness and relationality. I myself found this motivating when I worked as a GTA, in ways that Ingrid and Gretchen describe: even when I was tired, even when the students struggled or caused me discomfort, the moment when they would find my ovaries, cervix, or uterus for the first time brought me joy. Interviewing GTAs, they and I struggled to find language to talk about these moments. I made notes during my interviews of times when they and I would find ourselves simply saying "you know" to one another, and I *did* know. I find literatures on affect so helpful for understanding this almost radical connectivity: there was no way to describe these moments in language. It is simply an experience of shared feeling, between my GTA participants and me, between their students and them, between my students and me.

However, this should not be taken as evidence that GTAs' pleasure in intimacy is spontaneous and unstructured. Rather, it is part of the work that they perform. Sharing their joy over the intimate spaces of their bodies addresses "the quandary of the sacred vagina" (Posner 2015) in medical education: female reproductive anatomy has long held a taboo place in mainstream US culture and indeed in medicine (Barker-Benfield 2004). GTAs' work necessarily involves evoking pleasure and enjoying discovery in medical students who may not be predisposed to this kind of affective engagement. Even for students who come in curious, to use Gretchen's language, attending to and cultivating these affects are important for making certain kinds of physicians.

Likewise, GTAs cultivate specific and intuitive forms of intimacy with their coworkers based on these shared moments. This enables them to engage medical students in specific ways *and* it protects their bodies from potential harm. Grace, who is quoted at the beginning of this chapter, spoke of her comfort with working on and with the body of her training partner. She elaborated: "We support each other. We're fair with each other. There's an appropriate amount of humor. We're respectful to each other. I think we're protective of each other." Ingrid also spoke to this sense of camaraderie:

> It's really nice to know that there are other people . . . you can talk to about really funny things that happened during a session or . . . are you having a really hard time with . . . getting them to do the right levels of pressure [in the breast exam]? These are things I can't talk to my friends about that don't do this work. So I have a great support network of girl-friends, for instance, but when I told them I was going to this, they were like, well, that's kind of cool, but eww [*laughs*]. . . . So it's important to have the other GTAs that . . . have a more intimate understanding.

This understanding is in part about the shared bodily knowledge that GTAs develop. It is only logical to speak with coworkers who have also developed this knowledge about how to fine-tune their skills and use them to do this type of work. Ingrid appreciates asking for tips on how to translate her bodily experience (pressure) into something she can verbalize to students. But Ingrid hints at something larger that she gets from her relationship with her coworkers: forms of intimate under-standing, being able to laugh or commiserate about things that happen in a session. Ingrid's mention of her friends aligns with what I heard from many GTAs, which was that their loved ones supported the idea of their job but were somewhat dismayed by its exact details ("that's kind of cool, but eww").

Ingrid went on to describe the actual working relationship in the room, which involves intimacy and close knowledge of the work and each other's bodies:

> So . . . for instance . . . if I'm pre-menstrual, my breasts are much more sensitive and so getting the number of breast exams that I will be under-going can be fairly uncomfortable. . . . So your [GTA] partner may say, well, why don't I be the patient first . . . or, if she stays in the provider role, she may do a very light palpation herself. . . . If you're kind of at the very beginning or very end of your menstrual cycle, so there still could be blood in the vaginal canal, or still be blood present on the face of the cervix . . . it's really important that we communicate that with each other. . . . We try to make sure that they're [students] not squeamish or

uncomfortable, but we do take extra precaution. . . . We use gauze to kind of continuously clean off the . . . gloved hand of the student . . . and also hand our [GTA] partner gauze so that she can clean herself up so that she's more comfortable . . .

Ingrid described practices that several other GTAs told me about and that I myself observed or experienced while working as a GTA. GTAs have to communicate with each other about intimate changes to their bodies and work together based almost entirely on innate or unspoken coordination of efforts to keep the GTA on the table comfortable. GTAs who team-teach routinely touch each other's breasts or vulvas and see inside of each other's vaginas. Coworking relationships are deeply intimate. This is again necessary for this kind of affective labor: GTAs must simultaneously protect themselves and their bodies *and* manage the emotions of their students. Ingrid's partner needs to be aware of her menstrual cycle in order to protect Ingrid's comfort at the same time that she must be mindful of students' reactions to menstrual fluid.[13]

Jill likewise described the level of trust and attentiveness that GTAs who team-teach have to develop in order to do this work:

> The nature of the work that we do is such that we're really reliant on each other to be present and trust-worthy. . . . It is expected that the other person is available to help deal with anything that comes up. And also is the person who has a second set of eyes . . . on the room, on the instruments being cleaned, that the student is abiding by clean technique with their gloves and how they're handling instruments, whether they're touching anything else in the room and need to change their gloves, that kind of stuff. So there's a lot trust necessarily. It's a very intimate trust in that regard.

Jill speaks here of the intimate forms of coordination that occur as GTAs teach together that must occur to protect the health and safety of the GTA on the table. The GTA who takes the physician role has the task of being attentive over her partner's body in a unique way. She has to watch her partner at all times for signs of distress or unspoken communication about an issue that arises. At the same time, she keeps an eye on the students to keep the session moving along and keep the GTA on the table safe. Jill refers to the importance of cleanliness: because GTAs receive so many more pelvic exam than regular patients and because their work depends literally on the health of their vaginas, making sure that students observe clean technique is crucial. If a student touches a dusty tabletop or scratches their greasy nose before inserting a finger into the GTAs' vagina, that can cause health problems for the GTA that would put her out of work. The ability of GTAs to keep making money hinges on intimate attention between them and their partners. Or, if the GTA is working alone, intimate attention to the students' actions at all times.

Sticky Bodies in Intimate Labor

While intimacy is both a source of pleasure for GTAs and a resource necessary for their work, intimate labor can also open a worker up to perhaps greater intimacy than intended or to forms of intimacy beyond the worker's control. "Intimacy occurs in a social context; it is accordingly shaped by, even as it shapes, relations of race, class, gender, and sexuality" (Boris and Parreñas 2010:1). In this way, the intimate labor of GTAs is shaped primarily by gender and sexuality, since their work depends on their bodies. Cultural messages about bodies that are assigned female at birth associate them with sexuality, filth, and disorder.[14] These affects shape the experience of intimacy and paid labor for GTAs. Feminist theorist Sara Ahmed argues that emotions circulate in affective economies and gain value through their circulation (much in the way that money is valuable only because it is exchanged).[15] As signs—words or other forms of expression—circulate, they accumulate affects. These signs can become "sticky" or "saturated with affect" (Ahmed 2015:194) as "an effect of the histories of contact between bodies, objects, and signs" (Ahmed 2015:90). Sticky signs then become "stuck" to certain bodies, binding bodies to the emotions that circulate in social contexts.[16] In intimate labor, affective economies shape the experience of the work as individual workers attempt to manage this stickiness.

In my interviews with medical students, sex was the silent unspoken. While not all medical students may be uncomfortable, many are because this exam is so invasive and involves sexualized body parts. Medical students used words like "intimate" and "personal" to talk about the exam, and for many reasons that I discuss in the next chapter having to do with their nascent professional identities, I found it hard to get them to talk about why sexuality made them so uncomfortable. GTAs, however, were more able to speak about sexuality in reflexive and informative ways. While GTAs work very hard to maintain a desexualized space for the exam,[17] the moments when they struggle to uphold these boundaries often reveal insights into the stickiness of bodies.

Because of the importance of maintaining a desexualized intimate educational space, GTAs as a rule do not teach students with whom they have personal connections. Marie described an encounter when she agreed to teach a friend's partner, assuming that her professional boundaries would manage the situation, but experienced the intrusion of affect from elsewhere.

> It was a little bit weird because . . . it was slightly sexualized. . . . When they [the student] were doing my exam, they were intimate with my friend. . . . I couldn't help for it to be sexualized. . . . I couldn't help but thinking about this student and her interactions with my friend sexually. And then that being parallel with her interactions with me that were— could be mechanically similar. . . . Just her facial expressions were funny for some reason and I [wondered] if she made those same facial expressions when she was having sex.

In this way, unwanted affects are part of the GTA encounter because they have become stuck on the bodies of the medical students, in this case, through this student's sexual relationship with Marie's friend. However, they also become stuck to Marie's own body, through her experiences with affective economies of queer sex. For Marie, what made this encounter so uncomfortable was that her experiences of how her partners used their hands during sex were mimicked in the actions of the bimanual exam.

> The situation with this girl . . . she was cute and I like women. . . . You can have experiences as a GTA where you might have . . . some kind of at-traction to someone or it might be slightly sexualized. But as long as you draw that professional line and you don't act on it . . . I don't think there's anything wrong with that.

Other GTAs expressed similar experiences of finding themselves sexually attracted to the students. As Cassandra said, "A good-looking student walks into the room, and you kind of have to like rein your brain in a little bit." For this reason, part of the labor of that GTAs do involves managing this affective economy of sexuality and desire.

Gretchen described an encounter she had with two students in a way that more clearly highlights the role of how affects produced in economies of sexuality get stuck to bodies in GTA sessions.

> They were like sort of good-looking soccer jock kind of guys. I know it's all stereotypey [sic], but how they kind of registered in my mind. And Soccer Guy One finished with the speculum, took it out, looked at me in the face and said, "Thank you," and stepped to the side and said "Next!" in a way that looked totally out of a gang bang video.

Gretchen acknowledged that her students probably did not intend to invoke this particular arrangement of sexual practice in the encounter. Regardless, the situation resonated for her as one that evoked a specific form of heteronormative sexual culture. Gretchen described how she felt in that situation and what she saw as the parallel between that one encounter and that form of pornographic imagery:

> Part of what's going on there is . . . men having control of the woman's body, rather than the woman deciding singly who her sexual partners are going to be. So I had [a] sort of moment of like, so you're the students and you're passing me around like a textbook.

These affects were produced in affective economies of pornography and became stuck to Gretchen's body. In this way, disgust, shame, or degradation are affects that become bound to bodies assigned female at birth—even when sexuality is supposedly removed from the encounter. While this example may seem like an outlier, it demonstrates some connections and some departures from how the pelvic exam has historically been taught prior to the GTA program. The practice of multiple (male) medical students crowding around a woman's body to view her vagina "resembles a 'gang rape'" (Kapsalis 1997:64; see also Bell [2009:108]). Gretchen's use of the phrase "gang bang" indicates that some of the same affective economies of sexuality remain at work in teaching and learning the pelvic exam, with the difference now of a willing and consenting participant.

The very materiality of the body can sometimes introduce affective economies of sexuality into the GTA session, as was the case for Ingrid:

> I had intercourse . . . the night before, that was a little bit more . . . vigorous than maybe it should have been the day before I did a [teaching] session. And, so my body was reacting to that. . . . There was some redness and . . . it looked sort of like there'd been abrasions and whatnot.

For her, these visible markings indicated to her students and her teaching partner that she used her body for sexual pleasure as well as teaching. The conflicting sets of affects made her uncomfortable. She managed the situation by medicalizing her body:

> I could explain it away to them. This is ecchymosis. You know, I do have sensitive skin in this area, so this is normal for me, yada yada. But . . . I know that my face was flushing and I was uncomfortable, like I was letting them in on something in my private life that I wouldn't have ordinarily let strangers in on, but there wasn't any way sort of around it.

She framed the evidence of her sexuality on her body within a medical context, using the medical jargon of "ecchymosis" (that is, bruising), but the visible evidence nevertheless included her students her sexuality, which she otherwise kept separate from her teaching.

Ingrid's facial flushing and discomfort indicate feelings of shame, which aligns with larger societal expectations of women and sex. Gretchen likewise told me a story about how affective economies that ascribe shame to women's bodies shape how she experiences the teaching session.

> I'm always afraid that my feet stink. . . . Now I've kind of worked that in by making it a joke that, you know, women are really nervous about these exams for a lot of reasons. For example, I'm always nervous that my feet stink, it's not about you looking at my vagina. . . . I can do it to a certain

extent, but there are some body things that are still too personal for me to talk about with them.

Gretchen also spoke less directly about her feelings about other aspects of her body: "I think some of it's body shame. That I do think it's important for students to practice on fat women, but being a fat woman means body shame." Even though she liked the "radical politics that my queer fat body is the one that teaches how this goes," she still experienced feelings of vulnerability and even shame because she inhabits a fat body in a culture that devalues fatness—and medical culture does so especially.[18]

Thus, for paid workers who perform intimate labor, their work is shaped by gender, sexuality, race, class, and other social, cultural, and political structures, and these structures in term produce and are produced by circulations of affect. Intimate labor involves the management of stickiness, and GTAs must develop ways of maintaining their authority and setting barriers against unwanted intimacies.

Resisting Subordination in Intimate Labor

This discussion of how GTAs manage unintended affects that enter the session through affective economies of sexuality and gender leads me to some additional important points about the harms that GTAs face and how they manage these. Because of the work of managing affect and intimacy, and because of the potential for physical harm that they experience, GTAs must hone strategies for maintaining their authority and reducing the risks. This need underscores both the uniqueness of this kind of intimate labor and its kinship with other forms of bodily labor in which the worker's body is the site of work.[19]

While almost nothing done in a pelvic exam can cause lasting damage, and while the session is set up so that GTAs have full control over the actions done to their bodies, nearly all of the GTAs I interviewed voiced having experienced or being aware of a constant threat of bodily harm. Marie said: "The worst-case scenario really is . . . linked to [physical] discomfort . . . there wasn't a lot of emotional or psychological discomfort that I've experienced." Likewise, Ingrid stated the importance of controlling the students' actions: "You kind of have to really rein them in because at the end of the day, it's your body." Several educators described having the speculum "pop out," or be removed from the vagina while still fully opened, due to the inexperience or unwillingness of the student to follow direction. Other GTAs told stories about students whose nails had not been properly trimmed and who, as a result, scratched their vaginal walls. Sylvia recalled a student who "was really sort of overconfident in her knowledge and experience" and because of this "refused to close the speculum before she removed it" despite the explicit instruction to do so. In this way, in order to prevent bodily harm, GTAs must develop strategies for resisting subordination and maintaining authority.[20] These strategies are part of their repertoire of skills in intimate authority: negotiating control even in situations of extreme intimacy.

Some of these are taught during training, but most are learned through the experience of teaching the exam repeatedly. As Marie phrased it, "You learn in the moment and by thinking about and processing in that moment." As in other forms of intimate labor, the use of language and the regulation of touch are very important strategies. Students are given and follow explicit verbal commands as to what steps to take and how to perform the exam skills. Perhaps the most evident and immediate method of verbal control for GTAs is being able to tell the student to stop: as part of their training, GTAs are encouraged to tell students to stop or immediately change a physical behavior at any time if there is risk of harm. Most GTAs described situations in which they physically manipulated or stopped the student to prevent harm. Usually these situations involved difficulty with the speculum. As Anna explained, "I have on occasion reached down and held a student's hand to . . . make sure the speculum doesn't pop out with the bills still open." Likewise, Ingrid said: "I have literally stopped students in the middle of . . . the pelvic exam . . . particularly like inserting the speculum for instance. . . . I will physically take control of their hand or part of the instrument, help them float it out of my body. And then help to get them inserted more correctly and more comfortably." Thus, physical control is one of the primary methods that GTAs use. This strategy relies on careful and continual monitoring of the students and their physical behaviors in order to anticipate or correct problematic action.

In addition, most GTAs mentioned some form of management of their vocal tone in order to present themselves as professional and authoritative. Beth described this as "basic feminist communication theory," which includes not "end[ing] statements on an up tone or . . . sounding like you're questioning everything." She linked this approach to the gendered power dynamics of the encounter, rejecting "little things that women are frequently taught in communicating to seem less in control of things." Marie described her approach as "being able to . . . use a tone of voice that's . . . a little bit stern at times to establish that control." On the other hand, GTAs often use joking or humor to help relax nervous students and make them easier to work with. Grace uses "appropriate humor to kind of break the ice" if she believes that her students are very nervous. Beth finds the use of humor to be "mostly a matter of keeping the tone a little bit lighter. It really does help with the mood, with the students' stress levels, and most of them coming in are pretty stressed out." Ingrid's use of humor is in order to demonstrate for the students that she is "in control but in a nonthreatening way toward them." Some GTAs use the same jokes as part of their "script" to alleviate anxiety, diffuse tension, and to address student mistakes in a way that is nonthreatening. Vivian told me, "I just taught last night, and by the end of the session . . . we're all laughing and joking, you know, because it's like, oh, wow, you know, letting go." This use of humor stands in stark contrast to the sexist humor used by previous generations of medical faculty, which I describe in chapter 1. Humor is used in both of these contexts to forge social bonds: medical faculty attempted to enroll trainees in the "boys' club" of medicine by demeaning women, whereas GTAs use humor to help medical students let go of some anxiety and trust the GTAs' intimate authority.

Another technique that GTAs use to maintain their intimate authority is medicalized language. This demonstrates that their training involves studying some of the same materials that medical students study. Bonnie likes to "come across as super-informed" about anatomy and medical technologies because students may assume "we're less educated than we are." Vivian is an experienced educator who also is the coordinator for one of the programs in her area. She uses medical terminology because she wants the students to "know what [she's] specifically talking about like . . . the teres muscle or . . . lateral versus medial."[21] However, she also uses language to assert her authority when challenged. When she encountered a student who "thought [he] knew everything" because of his standing in medical school, she "just threw in a lot more medical jargon and, you know, gained his respect just through that."

In this way, tone, language, and physical control are all ways that GTAs resist subordination in the teaching encounter. However, GTAs also have strategies for resisting some of the forms of intimacy that can be too intimate or too close to themselves. These rely upon a separation of the self from the body in complicated ways. Because their work involves intimate and close attention, and because it relies upon their haptic knowledge of their own bodies, they must remain fully embodied during the teaching encounter. And yet, they are sharing their bodies with strangers, which can be threatening because of affective economies of sexuality—both for themselves and their students. In addition, in an interesting way, although they are teaching from their individual bodies, their bodies also stand in more broadly for *the* body of *the* patient. This shift in person and perspective was apparent in almost all of the interview transcriptions I reviewed.

I asked GTAs as part of my interview protocol to describe to me step by step how they teach the exam. Most of them gave instructions about how to do the exam referring to *the* body parts, instead of *their own* ("my") body parts. When I urged Anna in our follow-up interview to reflect more on this dynamic, she said:

> ANNA: It's kind of like in a way, teaching, there's maybe kind of part of us that steps aside because we have to kind of see things from their [students'] point of view . . . So it's kind of attributing to us, part of our consciousness and our vocalization, has to kind of be separate from being just in our body.
>
> KELLY: Do you think it's something that helps with the educational process or helps the GTA in any way?
>
> ANNA: It could be. It could be that it could make them feel more comfortable with it, that it feels less of an invasion in their privacy or their person. . . . I think in our culture, for most people, the area of their genitals and breasts tends to be an area of high privacy . . . so that might help them kind of distance it or make it feel like okay, so right now, it's not *me* that they're examining. It's the body as a tool, as a device to help them learn.

Anna reports using this language herself sometimes for the comfort of the students, but she also reflects on the idea of the genitals as being "areas of high privacy," parts of the body that, for some people, are too intimate to be shared with strangers. The language shift both allows GTAs to take on the students' perspective and reduce the intimacy of the experience for themselves. Likewise, Vivian said:

> I know that I've caught myself actually saying, you know, I'm talking third-person or something like that and it seems really weird to me. I think it depersonalizes it for the students, so it becomes easier if they want to have a conversation about something that's very personal with the person that they're actually working with. . . . It's not *me* anymore, it's *the* cervix, or you know what I mean? (Emphasis added.)

Vivian accounts here for her use of third-person language as being for the students' comfort. Sylvia likewise located the language shift in the attempt to protect another person's comfort, in this case, her teaching partner's: "I think that it would probably be an effort to kind of reduce any embarrassment . . . that maybe the person would feel like . . . it's a more objective experience. Like you don't have to be concerned about embarrassing this person." She went on to say that she dislikes teaching in pairs because she sometimes feels excluded from the educational experience because of these dynamics.

In our follow-up interview, Marie and I had an interesting exchange about the different contexts in which other people touch her cervix and how she relates to them and her body in such moments.

> MARIE: I guess it's just about me using my body as a model . . . when I'm talking to a partner, I would use *my*, but when I'm teaching, I would use *the*. And it's interesting because I think it kind of depersonalizes it for me.
>
> KELLY: And what do you mean when you say it depersonalizes it?
>
> MARIE: So, it makes it less intimate, you know, like if I'm talking to a partner and I'm saying, "Look . . . feel . . . this is my cervix." It's more of like an intimate experience, like they're touching *me*, whereas for whatever reason when I'm working with students . . . I don't want that to be so intimate . . . so I say *the* because . . . I tend to make

myself more like a model. . . . They are touching me, they're definitely touching me, but the language I use . . . makes it less intimate.

KELLY: So the role then of the . . . language that you use is . . . to make it a less intimate experience between you and your students? Is that what I'm hearing you say?

MARIE: Yes . . . it professionalizes it. . . . And do you know what's interesting, too, is . . . recently like a couple weeks ago, me and a couple different women did like an informal . . . see your cervix session. And I definitely used the language *my*. . . . it was more of like an informal like friends of friends thing and they were not students. . . . I noticed that that experience was very different from working with students as a GTA, because . . . I felt that I was comfortable being less professional.

Even though Marie approaches GTA work as an empowering experience of sharing her body, she is also aware of the intimacy that such work involves. As our exchange demonstrates, the meaning of intimate forms of bodily contact vary based on context. All intimacy is not paid labor, and not all intimate labor is necessary paid, as her informal workshop with friends demonstrates (Zelizer 2010). Language, then, allows GTAs to actively shape the context of their paid intimate labor and to *professionalize* such forms of visceral contact.

Intimacy, then, is always already prestructured by its social, cultural, and economic contexts. It is shot through with affective economies that stick some bodies and body parts to some emotions more than others. GTAs use a variety of techniques for maintaining authority in encounters that could otherwise render them subordinate. Even their use of the article "the," rather than the pronoun "my," manages just how intimate their intimate authority is.

New Forms of Work in Medical Education

Intimate labor produces many forms of value (Boris and Parreñas 2010; Mankekar and Gupta 2016; Vora 2010; Zelizer 2005). When such labor is affective, as GTA work is, it does so through the circulation of affect (Vora 2010). This labor of course produces economic value through the accumulation or manipulation of affects. For GTAs, this value is the relatively high hourly pay that they receive, while for corporatized healthcare this is the money made from physicians who are empathetic and rate highly in measures of patient-satisfaction. However, intimate labor that is affective also produces other kind of values: new forms of sociality, connectivity, and community. This kind of labor produces new subjectivities, especially in the case of education labor. Indeed, intimate labor produces biopower when it is affective. By *biopower*, I mean a uniquely modern form of power over biological life, through which "lives may be managed on both an individual and a group basis" (Taylor 2011:44). Put more simply, intimate labor denotes a kind of labor that produces power over the management of lives.

Michael Hardt argues for conceptualizing biopower from below through his analysis of affective labor, according to which the purpose of affective labor is the creation of value under these new modes of capitalist production (1999). As such, affective labor is the work of creating forms of connectivity, sociality, and community. It is the work of creating connections between different human beings in the service of capitalism. Exemplary types of work include call-center representatives, healthcare workers, and nannies (Ducey 2010; Mankekar and Gupta 2016; Twigg 2000; Vora 2010). These are all types of work that do not produce a tangible item but still keep the gears of capitalism running. They are also all feminized and precarious forms of work, often part-time or flexible, without benefits such as health insurance or retirement plans. Likewise, in healthcare, sociologist Ariel Ducey has explored "soft skills" training programs for healthcare workers that focused on "customer service, communication skills, team building and teamwork, cultural diversity, conflict resolution, and leadership training" (2010:24). Ducey links these programs and this massive reskilling of health care workers in the 1990s to broader shifts from discipline to control and the reorganization of the economy around forms of immaterial labor. Given that care and caring for patients are central to the work of nurses, nurse aids, and even, increasingly, physicians, technologies of affect such as those that Ducey has described and those that I analyze in this book are intended to create more productive workers, workers more useful to capital and empire.

I use this as a jumping off point to think about the labor that GTAs do in medical education—and that simulated patients do more broadly. These are forms of affective labor aimed not at the production and modulation of affect(s), but at the production of sociality, community, and, indeed, biopower. The work that GTAs and simulated patients do is about producing future physicians who connect with their patients, communicate well, empathize. Their work is about the production of new subjectivities—through the socialization of the next generation of medical students. And, thus, their work also produces biopower by creating new physicians who can operate in new regimes of affect in healthcare, in which the production of "life itself" (Rose 2009) dominates over the prevention or treatment of disease. GTAs and other simulated patients work to create experts who can more effectively manage the conduct of populations in new landscapes of patient consumerism and corporatized healthcare.

This is a radically new form of work in medical education, with a radically new type of workforce. It is an industry that has sprung up since the 1980s and generates a large economic footprint.[22] One medical school reported spending $20,000 per year on administrative costs, training, and hourly rates for GTAs (Jacques 2003) while another reported approximately $14,500 (Janjua et al. 2018).[23] While this is not a large part of medical school budgets, it demonstrates an ongoing financial investment. Another study placed the cost of using simulated patients to teach about 150 medical students physical exam skills at $43,800 for two years, including simulated patient and administrator pay (Hasle, Anderson, and Szerlip 1994).[24] And this is to say nothing of the cost of building and running a facility equipped to do simulated patient exams. This is a precarious but specially skilled new workforce that produces new forms of governmentality in medicine by crafting more sensitive, more empathetic physicians. This has profound consequences for the future of work in healthcare and the production of value out of health, illness, and the clinic. I take these themes up more fully in the next chapter.

4

Practicing Professionalism, Performing Authenticity

In 2010, not long before I started formulating the research project that would eventually become this book, the University of Minnesota Medical School generated controversy by eliminating its gynecological teaching associate program in favor of plastic manikins. An article in *Inside Higher Ed* quoted the associate dean for curriculum and evaluation as saying that "we would never decide something just based on money," but the article's author was quick to point out that the school spends $150,000 every year training and paying simulated patients: "The change will probably save at least a few thousand dollars" (Epstein 2010). Medical students, patients, and physicians at other institutions criticized the move (Bannow 2010; Kesti 2010; Pho 2010). These critics all agreed that there is something about the pelvic exam that cannot be taught on a manikin; it must be taught on the actual person receiving it. Even Carla Pugh, a physician who invented one of the most sophisticated manikins available (used by over one hundred medical schools), was skeptical of the decision: "I've never promoted mannequin-based [sic] trainers as a replacement for standardized patients. . . . In my teaching, I have used a combined approach using mannequins, the simulator and patients" (Epstein 2010).[1] The senior director for educational affairs at the Association of American Medical Colleges, M. Brownell Anderson, defended the use of manikins: "The mannequins [sic] allow them [medical students] to practice over and over and over again" (Bannow 2010). Jane Zanutto Crone, a professor at the University of Wisconsin School of Medicine and Public Health affirmed the importance of GTAs. "You will never be in the situation again where you go to palpate someone's ovary and they say, 'You're nowhere near it. Let me tell you how to move your hand.' . . . A true patient is not going to give you that kind of feedback" (Bannow 2010).

One thing that these comments address is the precariousness of GTA work, which I have discussed in the previous chapter. When budgets are constrained, these programs are more likely to be first on the chopping-block. GTAs know that there is no guarantee that they will be asked to teach the following year by any given medical school. And yet, these comments also suggest that the performance of the pelvic exam isn't entirely about the manual or technical skill of the exam. There is value in GTAs' labor that a manikin cannot replicate, as medical students themselves recognize. Thus, for example, the *Inside Higher Ed* article on the University of Minnesota, noted that a

> fourth year [student], John Thomas Egan, said he and his classmates consider the practice exam "an important learning tool, taking students who perhaps may never have been involved with any sort of intimate exam or touch and giving them this experience in a very safe space." The initial one-on-one interaction with a patient who's comfortable with her body is helpful in calming nerves and building confidence, Egan added. "As a guy, at least, there's a certain amount of anxiety" about conducting a pelvic exam. (Epstein 2010)

Writing on the importance of GTA sessions, obstetrician Adam Wolfberg also emphasizes that there is more to the exam than mere manual skill. "Students and professors say that for an examination that can be painful and embarrassing, it is invaluable to have someone reflect on the patient's experience while providing guidance and instruction" (Wolfberg 2007).

This debate highlights several things. Medical students need practice to become proficient, and yet practicing on actual clinic patients has become controversial. Manikins are helpful, but do not adequately address the emotions that go along with doing such an intimate exam for the first time. Simulation is increasingly sophisticated and simulated patients have important skills; that is what makes these programs costly. These tensions underscore concern among faculty in medical education about the best or most appropriate way to train the next generation of physicians, as I've discussed in chapter 2. They also signal the entangled nature of manual skills with emotion in the pelvic exam: being a good physician is about much more than being able to locate and palpate a cervix. There is something dispositional here as well. Or, more accurately, there is something affective—something that simulation with real people prepares trainees differently than simulation with manikins.

In this chapter, I am concerned with how it is that "fake" encounters with GTAs and other simulated patients can produce "real" physicians. By a real physician, I mean someone who thinks, acts, talks, and feels like a competent, confident physician. It is widely recognized that simulation plays an important part in medical student socialization (Harter and Kirby 2004; Prentice 2013; Vinson 2019). And yet the mechanisms of socialization remain understudied, and almost no attention has been paid to the affective dimensions of professional socialization via simulation.[2] I argue that the GTA session serves as a crucial step in the emotional socialization of medical students. I explore the tensions between artificiality and authenticity in order to understand how medical students come to embody medical culture through the pedagogical work that occurs in simulation. In this way, I consider simulation as a type of technology of affect proliferating in contemporary medical education and show how simulation produces medical subjects who learn to experience and manage emotion in ways that align with the dominant discourses in biomedicine.[3]

Simulation as a Technology of Affect

In order to become a "real" physician, medical students undergo a prolonged training period in which they must learn how to navigate the unfamiliar attitudes, behaviors, rituals, specialized knowledge, institutional hierarchies, and so on, of the medical profession (Becker 2002). The concept of *habitus* is useful for making sense of how medical students come to embody medical culture, which "teaches doctors ways of negotiating their identities within the medical hierarchy and structure" (Luke 2003:xiii). French sociologist Pierre Bourdieu developed his concept of habitus to refer to the ways in which the individual is unconsciously oriented to a given field. Habitus is "understood as a system of lasting, transposable dispositions which, integrating past experiences, functions at every moment as a matrix of perceptions, appreciations, and actions" (Bourdieu 1977:83). Habitus is (1) acquired, (2) operates below the level of conscious awareness, (3) varies by social location, and (4) results from pedagogical work (Bourdieu 1977, 2000; Wacquant 2014a, 2014b). Scholars have found the concept of the habitus useful for understanding how embodied identities are shaped and transformed by broader terrains of power, as well as processes of resistance and change (Crossley and Crossley 2001; Decoteau 2013; Gould 2009; McNay 1999).

The concept of *habitus* was originally developed by Bourdieu to describe durable dispositions instilled in the subject without awareness or intention during childhood. However, in his later work on habitus, Bourdieu differentiated the generic habitus from the specific habitus. The specific habitus encompasses those dispositions that are "gradually, progressively and imperceptibly" (Bourdieu 2000:11) transformed after intentional entry into a given, more specialized field. Building upon Bourdieu's work, his student Loïc Wacquant adopts the terms "primary" and "secondary" habitus instead. I rely on Wacquant's definition of the secondary (or specific) habitus: "any system of transposable schemata that becomes grafted subsequently, through specialized pedagogical labor that is typically shortened in duration, accelerated in pace, and explicit in organization" (Wacquant 2014a:7). According to Wacquant, the greater the distance between the generic (or primary) habitus and the secondary (or specific) habitus, "the more difficult the traineeship, and the greater the gaps and frictions between the successive layers of schemata, the less integrated the resulting dispositional formation is likely to be" (Wacquant 2014a:8). Wacquant's work is particularly useful here for understanding the pedagogical work of inculcating the habitus, which involves the deliberate repetition of actions of the body until they fade from awareness and become a "natural" or unconscious facet of embodiment.

I draw from conceptualization of the secondary habitus to understand what scholars have called the "medical habitus" (Brosnan 2009, 2010; Lempp 2009; Luke 2003; Sinclair 1997). Sociologist Caragh Brosnan (2009, 2010) has extended Bourdieu's work to develop a framework for the relationship between institutional arrangements in medicine and student practices or cultures. The durability of the field of medicine as it is structured and the reproduction of medical habitus help explain both the valuing of "competence" over caring in medical education and the "reform without change" effected by curricular transformation. Using the concept of the medical habitus allows scholars to move beyond purely cognitive models of socialization to consider the transformation of thoughts, perceptions, feelings, and modes of embodiment of medical students as they adapt to medical culture (Prentice 2013). As a secondary habitus, the medical habitus also equips its practitioners for close, intimate, or invasive contact with strangers' bodies (Giuffre and Williams 2000; Underman 2011). For example, anthropologist Rachel Prentice draws from conceptualizations of habitus in her ethnography of surgical training in medical school to understand how trainees adapt to "touching, invading, and sometimes doing violence to patients' bodies in the name of healing" (2013:65). In this way, the medical habitus is a useful concept for understanding the process of subject-formation in medical training.

One of the core tensions of the medical habitus is often that competency displaces caring (Brosnan 2009; Sinclair 1997). Medical students and physicians alike have difficulty reconciling the scientific disposition required of medicine with their idealistic notions of caring and compassion. Studies of medical schools have shown that medical students enter with a desire to care for patients and reduce human suffering and leave feeling cynical and depersonalizing their patients. The adoption of a cynicism is a response to the institutional pressures of the hospital and the emotionally taxing work of dealing every day with suffering and death (Becker 2002). In addition, important rituals such as working with cadavers in the anatomy lab socialize medical students to discard feelings of fear, disgust, or horror, to view patients as body-objects (Hafferty 1988; Smith and Kleinman 1989), and thereby to cultivate an attitude of "detached concern" (Fox 1979).[4] While the literature on emotional socialization in medical school makes it seem as though emotion is being socialized *out of* medical students through this shift from compassion to competence, I claim instead that competence is itself an affective disposition, a particular way of feeling embedded in a cultural context.

As I show, simulation is one type of mechanism for practicing affective dispositions. In his ethnography of a boxing club, sociologist Steve Hoffman argues that simulations "are those repeatable activities that are defined by members of a task group as an approximation of some other scenario or activity that is more real" (2006:175). Participants in simulation engage in what Hoffman calls "everyday ontology": belief that the simulation is analogous to a real situation means that the consequences of a simulation are real. For Hoffman, simulation serves three functions. First, simulation is about risk-management. Second, simulation helps foster professional socialization because it is one way in which "practitioners . . . try out different techniques, behaviors, and social roles that may or may not be adopted later" (Hoffman 2006:174). Third, simulations are flexible and transportable, in that they "are simplified subsets of a more complicated reality" (Hoffman 2006:176). Breaking reality down into these subsets of skills and actions allows such skills and actions to be taken across a variety of social situations and physical spaces.

It is my contention that the low-risk, ontologically flexible, and playful nature of simulation makes it beneficial for overcoming the gap between the generic and specific habitus. As Wacquant argues, the larger the gap between the generic and the specific habitus, the harder it will be for the trainee to fully inculcate the secondary habitus. The artificiality of the GTA session makes consequences not as serious, which helps the trainee try out—and begin to embody—the dispositions of the unfamiliar cultural context, meaning clinical medicine. Furthermore, it is my contention that because part of the conflict between the primary and secondary habitus in medical school is about emotion (as in, the conflict between caring and competence), it is the emotional resonance (or lack thereof) of the simulation in the GTA session that dictates how successful or unsuccessful it will be in the long-term inculcation of the medical habitus. For the successful inculcation of a secondary habitus, it does not matter that the simulation is not real if it *feels* real.

Practicing Professionalism in Simulation

Coming into medical school, many students have no idea of how to behave. As Molly, a medical student, described:

> There were several students on first day of our surgery rotation who'd never stepped into a surgery. And so if you don't know what the atmosphere of the operating room was like, what you can touch or you can't touch, what's sterile, what's not, how to scrub in, who to talk to, what to tell them, the operating room can be a really scary place and uncomfortable for us students. There's people who do this every day. So this is second nature to them. . . . And so that's mysterious for us [medical students].

Molly's description of surgery is an excellent example of the ways in which normal, commonsense behaviors and dispositions no longer work in the clinical setting. Basic tasks such as washing your hands or how and when to speak to other people become imbued with new rules and norms. Behaviors such as touching or not touching now carry literal life and death significance (since all of the extremely stringent rules about hygiene in surgery are for a very good reason: preventing deadly infections). Molly's description also underscores the affective dimension of the experience: the operating room is *scary and uncomfortable*. Molly went on to connect this to the pelvic exam:

> In a similar way, I think the gynecological exam is kind of a black box, a thing that you know physicians do and you know you're probably going to have to do it. And I think if I've never seen it, oh, shit! I'm going to have to perform this on someone.

For medical students, watching a resident or physician perform the exam on a patient can make it seem like a black box; all of the experiential knowledge, perception, and judgment and the comfort with the sensitive nature of the exam are hidden inside the body of the experienced physician. Hence, the growth of simulation: medical students need to see and do the same things as experienced physicians to uniformly prepare them for the profession.

In this way, understanding milestones is important for opening the black box of medical socialization. The medical students I interviewed often spoken of these moments as learning *professionalism*, a term they used over and over again in interviews to refer to a set of practices including verbal and nonverbal communication and attitudes that signified a "real" physician.[5] The goal of professionalism and consciously developing professional skills is to eventually be able to think, act, and feel (in a triple sense: experience emotion, tactile sense, sense of oneself) like a physician without having to deliberately reflect on the appropriate behavior. Thus, simulation is a terrain in which medical students can try out the skills, values, and attitudes that they have been learning about and discussing in the classroom.

The GTA session is an important example of the way in which simulation produces certain kinds of medical subjectivities. Like encountering cadavers in the anatomy lab, the experience of learning the pelvic exam requires medical students to manage their initial emotional reaction (Fox

1979; Hafferty 1988). However, the pelvic exam in today's medical education involves far more than simply learning to suppress unprofessional emotions. It involves a range of skills and techniques to both present oneself as a knowledgeable and compassionate physician *and* make the patient comfortable (and thus foster desirable emotions in the patient).

The students I interviewed spoke about performing the pelvic exam as an important rite in their education, as the first time they would have to touch an actual, living person in a sensitive and sexually charged area of the body without reacting negatively. As Jacob said, "When you do this, the [pelvic] exams, it just feels like you're in medical school." While medical students practice parts of the head-to-toe exam on simulated patients prior to working with GTAs, for the majority of them, the GTA encounter is the first time they will touch genitals in a clinical setting. Consequently, the stakes of professionalism are heightened. As Ellie said, "These [pelvic] exams are sort of personal. . . . They are sensitive exams by definition . . . [and] such extensive exams require a slightly higher level of professionalism." The skillset of "professionalism" includes managing the emotional states or anxieties that the pelvic exam can evoke. As Molly put it, "If you're nervous, the patient can tell, so I think that's [the GTA session] a valuable experience." Michelle described professionalism as "projecting confidence even if I don't feel confident." Learning to project this competence and confidence is essential for medical socialization, and it leads to embodying these values as the medical students inculcate the medical habitus.

Professionalism is also crucial for maintaining barriers while working on another's body (Hafferty 1988; Lempp 2009). The associated skillsets shape the medical student's emotions during the exam, as well as the patient's, such as the "ICE" mnemonic ("inspect," "check," "examine") that I discuss in chapter 3. The medical students I spoke with seemed to really internalize these lessons about language as an important marker of their professionalism. Ellie explained:

"Feel" is a word that can elicit sort of emotional feelings when you're performing an exam. . . . Patients are probably more primed to hear something like that and have it eliciting confused or emotional response during a sensitive exam. . . . Exams are all about the communication between doctor and the patient.

Ellie's discussion of clinical language here underscores her sense of pride in being able to navigate the pelvic exam with acumen. For medical students like Ellie, mastering the nuances of language demonstrated their progress on the pathway from novice to expert.

They felt that they *appeared* to be competent, confident professionals, even if they didn't fully embody competence and confidence yet. Regardless, professional language could influence the patient's experience. As Ellie noted, a student should avoid "eliciting [a] confused or emotional response" while performing a pelvic exam. In this way, the skills of professional socialization serve a dual function: even as they shape the medical student's sense of self, they also shape the patient's experience.

Another skillset of professionalism is learning to manage touch. In chapter 3, I gave the example of Marie's struggle to professionalize forms of touch, which is a delicate process. Learning how to touch (or how not to touch) a patient fashions medical students into certain kinds of physicians, who are concerned about comfort, modesty, and so forth. These techniques are meant to make patients feel safe and trusting of the physicians. GTAs teach students how to wash their hands and put on gloves with clean technique (which reduces the amount of bacteria, viruses, or dust in an exam room that can be transferred to the vagina via the hands). Handwashing reduces disease transmission, but it is also an important signal to patients that the physician is concerned about the patient's health and wellbeing.[6] Likewise, GTAs teach medical students how to appropriately drape and undrape the patient. As medical student Stephanie said:

> There's a lot of sensitive things that are priority in the doctor-patient relationship . . . [like] creating modesty and just keeping the right amount of a patient's body uncovered . . . That's something you can do always, even if you're just working on someone's lung and that would make people feel more comfortable.

In this way, learning to manage the drape helps medical students acquire a disposition of sensitivity and concern for the patient's wellbeing, even at the same time as managing the drape is intended to produce or provoke comfort in the patient.

As Stephanie's remark demonstrates, these dispositions are not specific to the GTA session. Learning how to manage language, touch, and draping in any exam context was one of the most frequent replies when I asked medical students whether they had learned anything from the GTA encounter that would be applicable beyond the exam. As Jacob said, the GTA session "gave me a peek into all of the stuff that goes into a medical education. . . . They're [the GTAs] trying to shape you as a doctor." For Jacob and other students who answered similarly, while the GTA session is ostensibly about clinical skills for the pelvic exam, it is also about "shap[ing] you as a doctor." It is one stage among many that seeks to transform medical students' embodiment. Roger likewise said:

> Learning to talk to the patients and let them know what you are doing, so that they know what to expect . . . I think that is helpful and it's not just applicable to these sensitive exams. If you are putting an IV in somebody and you don't warn them, they are going to jump but if you tell them, hey you are going to feel a poke, so then they know to expect it. . . . That is something that is transferable. . . . The more experience you have examining patients, the better you get and the more comfortable you are.

Here, practicing the skills of the pelvic exam leads to a greater *sense of comfort* about dealing with patients in general. In this way, the GTA session aligns with other forms of simulation, as I discuss in chapter 2. Many of the aspects of performing a pelvic exam, such as examining patients with confidence and learning how to communicate about the exam, are applicable to other clinical contexts. Taken together, "professionalism" can be understood as a range of attitudes *and* actions that signify a "real" physician, meaning that professionalism is a component of the medical habitus. It is a set of values, dispositions, and behaviors that align the medical student with the culture of medicine. By deliberately rehearsing a specific set of skills linked to professionalism in the GTA session, medical students begin to lay the groundwork for embodying this culture.

Medical students recognized that professionalism is a skill that cannot be learned out of a book. It must be learned situationally, in a context where they are forced to interact with a real, live person. Medical student Sarah explained:

[Clinical skills education classes] try to . . . teach you professionalism and I think it's something that can't necessarily be taught. . . . You have to like learn it by experience. . . . You can't really teach professionalism. You can say what you should do, but until you're in a situation, like sort of teach by example I guess.

Medical students told me rather frequently that they were not sure if they could embody professionalism until they were in the room with a living person and had to perform an exam. This highlights the hands-on nature of the work of inculcating the medical habitus: it must be rehearsed quite literally in the flesh.

Medical students at one of the schools I studied were very protective of their emerging culture of medical professionalism. Several mentioned the following story as a violation of this culture. Tricia described it to me mostly clearly:

Somebody in our class made a joke [on Facebook] about the exam, and it was like very inappropriate and unprofessional. . . . He says like, "Doing my breast exam on Valentine's Day, guaranteed play." . . . I think he's not realizing that by putting that on Facebook . . . if one of his friends [. . . sees it . . .] and his friend is going for a breast exam tomorrow, and then she's like, "Wait a minute, is my doctor like thinking like this is play?"

This medical student's joke made an association between performing the breast exam and a sexual situation ("getting play"). Even though the joke was made in the semiprivate, nonprofessional context of Facebook, it threatened the emerging culture of professionalism that the students were developing by sexualizing the work that physicians and GTAs do. This student's comment also harkens back to 1970s feminist critiques that I discuss in chapter 1 and the resulting shift *away* from the acceptability of this kind of blatant "boys club" humor. The norms of professionalism have indeed changed: the students themselves responded; the class president sent out stern emails reminding students to remain professional in every context. Thus, professionalism isn't simply part of on-the-job work, but rather it relates to the larger (changing) field of clinical medicine and one's place within it. Medical students aren't just training to practice medicine like a physician—they are training to think, act, and *be* physicians, which is a transformation in identity that doesn't stop at the clinic doors.

This story is also important because of what it represents about medical students' relationship to sexuality in the context of the pelvic exam. In my interviews with them, sexuality was never explicitly mentioned or was mentioned only in roundabout ways as a potential threat to be removed from the encounter. Their lack of discussion about their own sexual feelings—even when I probed them to more fully explain *why* they felt uncomfortable doing the pelvic exam—demonstrates how even in the first or second year of medical school the need to desexualize intimate contact (or at least appear to, to a relative stranger conducting the interview) has become embodied. GTAs, on the other hand, were far more willing to open up about the slippages in sexuality during the pelvic exam, as I discuss in chapter 3.[7]

Thus, the GTA session is an important component of developing professionalism as part of inculcating the medical habitus. Medical education shares a lot in common with Wacquant's (2004) example of training a boxer. It involves an intentional repetition of actions and attitudes until these become unconsciously part of the body and psyche. Rehearsing the acts associated with professionalism, by learning to control touch, words, and emotions, leads to adopting professionalism as second nature. As I show, simulation helps medical students inculcate the medical habitus by allowing them to rehearse the skills and attitudes required of a competent professional physician in a low-stakes environment. These skills and attitudes are transportable and flexible and can be used in arenas of patient care outside of the pelvic exam.

Benefits of Simulation

As I discuss in chapters 1 and 2, due to ethical shifts and the declining length of hospital stays in the 1970s, medical students no longer use their skills for the first time on actual clinical patients. Rather, they rehearse them through the low-risk environment of simulation. This was a theme I heard commonly from medical faculty. For example, MD faculty member Miriam told me: "By the time you get to the patient, you know how to do it, you did most of your mistakes already." Such mistakes are not limited to poor technique improper use of instruments. They can be affective, too: embarrassing themselves or the patient is often one of the strongest fears that medical students have about the pelvic exam. For this reason, practicing first in a low-risk environment is important.

Students expressed over and over in my interviews that they appreciated being able to try out and gain some mastery of the skills that they would be expected to perform in the clinical setting. Students are aware of the risks to themselves and to patients, and they want the chance to try out the techniques first. The students I spoke with found it especially important to be able to practice their skills on a living person who would not rush them or otherwise be too uncomfortable. Medical student Jeff put it this way:

> I feel like with the [GTA] teacher, you can explore as much as you like. With a patient, you can explore, but you run the risk of like, why is his [the medical student's] hand still there. . . . With the [GTA], you can do as much as you want, as little as you want, whatever. With the patient . . . you're there until you find what you need to find, then you're done.

For Jeff and other medical students who echoed his viewpoint, the GTA allows them an opportunity to explore the performance of clinical skills, including the technical-manual exam skills and the communication or interpersonal interaction skills. This type of simulation removes the techniques that medical students are attempting to master from the explicitly goal-oriented actions of the clinic. What this means is that the GTA session allows medical students more time and more freedom for reflection and exploration. This reflexivity is a crucial component of simulation, as it leads to a remaking of the medical students' subjectivity. The extant literature in medical education also bears out this finding.[8]

A number of medical students told me that they were apprehensive about examining real patients because of the limited amount of feedback they might receive. The GTA session reduces risk by allowing for freer and more open communication about technique and potential harm. As medical student Roger explained:

> Let's just say I were doing a speculum exam on a patient and there was the head physician behind me and I am inserting it wrong and I don't know if the physician would be willing to say something like, hey you know if you

do that you can slice your urethra and cause trauma to the patient. That will make the patient I think kind of nervous and upset.

While the pelvic exam is on the whole very safe, there are still some risks of bruising, tearing, and damage to the genitals and reproductive organs. Simulation through the use of GTAs reduces physical harm to actual patients from the inexperienced behaviors or mistakes of medical students and thus improves patient care.

Moreover, simulation also reduces emotional risk—both for students and for patients. Students often experience a great deal of anxiety about the pelvic exam, both because of the intimate nature of the exam and the fear of patient contact more broadly. Nervousness could lead to mistakes that might harm the patient physically, which is why practicing in a simulation encounter protects patients. And yet, as Roger's statement also indicates, simulation reduces risk to student and patient by managing the emotional impact of mistakes on the student. It is noteworthy that while Roger's hypothetical supervisor was concerned about "slicing the urethra," Roger's own concerns were about making the patient "nervous and upset" by hearing that. Likewise, Michelle said:

> I was really nervous . . . [The exam is] very sensitive and [it's] not one that as a patient you look forward to having. So I was nervous about sort of doing that as a first year med student and having no experience, no expertise but sort of acting kind of presumptuous enough to perform them on actual people.

This comment reflects what I noticed overall in my interviews with medical students about performing the pelvic exam for the first time on a living person. They reported feeling nervous about appearing to not know what they were doing, about hurting the patient, and about having to touch someone in such an intimate area for the first time. Daphne said:

> The anxiety that everyone had was like a baseline anxiety. . . . I feel like it's [the GTA session] less about learning and perfecting the technique early but more just like practice or like doing something that's uncomfortable, like confronting the anxiety and making yourself and the patient comfortable.

The GTA experience thus allowed medical students a comfortable, safe environment to rehearse their skills, and led to a reduction in their anxiety about performing the exam. A number of studies back up this finding, as I outline in chapter 2 (Ziv et al. 2003). However, Daphne's statement also demonstrates the intersubjective nature of the emotion management skills that medical students acquire in the GTA session. Both students and patients have feelings about the exam. Through simulation, students learn how to manage both sides of this relationship.

The skills that students acquire through simulation are flexible and transportable. Students found the experience valuable not just for performing the pelvic exam, but in general for learning about patient contact. Molly explained: "I think as medical students . . . we're constantly walking into situations that we've never experienced before and things that we're not entirely comfortable with. So to cut out some of the mystery of examining the patient . . . in a clinical setting . . . the better off we are." The medical students I interviewed who voiced a similar opinion appreciated the GTA session because it was perhaps the most intimate and intense patient-contact experience they had in their first or second year of medical school. While the skills they learned were beneficial for the pelvic exam, having performed an exam that was so intimate and had such a potential to be awkward allowed them to conquer this hurdle of being nervous about any sort of bodily contact with patients. This is why I claim that the GTA session prepares medical students to embody the medical habitus: the flexibility and transportability of the skills developed in simulation become part of the overall disposition of a "real" physician. Uncertainty is a fact of life in medical culture, which means that the medical habitus must equip its practitioner with the tools to adjust to any situation they encounter.

A major component of the medical habitus is being able to attend to the patient experience. As medical student Carolina explained:

> You can do that by sitting around and talking about what the patients might think or how we as physicians feel when we are patients or when our families are patients, but . . . the more you can actually elicit patient . . . feedback . . . that's like the closest to authentic way to . . . aid our developing mentality of being . . . really aware of the patient experience and

attentive to the patient experience and I think that's more of an authentic way to kind of like to create patient-centered doctors . . . even if they're not quite a real patient.

Medical faculty, students, and GTAs themselves all voiced similar opinions about the benefits of using GTAs to teach the pelvic exam. These benefits went beyond performing the pelvic exam, and all three groups of stakeholders whom I interviewed credited GTAs with teaching students to be mindful of patient experiences in general. Despite students' awareness that these situations are artificial, such encounters provided a more "authentic way" of centering the patient experience. While this was at times related to a desire to empathize with patients, in interviews with faculty and students it was more often connected to the professional skills a medical student must master to be seen as competent by colleagues and patients. Thus, awareness of a patient does not necessarily mean appreciating the patient's subjectivity, but it is linked to a range of techniques that medical students must learn as part of developing the medical gaze (Foucault 1994).

Simulation of the pelvic exam through GTA sessions is especially beneficial for medical schools because the sessions have been more or less standardized, as I discuss in chapters 1 and 2. As PhD medical faculty member Elaine explained: "One of the things it [simulation] allows is for students . . . to get a consistent experience." This consistency is achieved in part by the use of scripts and checklists (see Appendix B). Lena, a program coordinator who runs several of the GTA programs that I studied, told me that she frequently checks in with her GTAs to make sure that they are all teaching the same material in a consistent manner. What this means is that rather than having medical students gain their skills from a single or select group of physicians, who may have individualized approaches and practices, GTAs make certain that medical students learn the same set of skills.

Thus, simulation offers a chance to rehearse the skills required of physicians in a low-risk environment. This skillset is what my participants and I have referred to as "professionalism": a range of attitudes and actions that signify a competent, confident physician. Professionalism is a part of the medical habitus, which must be rehearsed to be fully embodied. Simulation allows medical students to "play" at being physicians as they *become* physicians. Or, in other words, simulation works to inculcate the medical habitus. This is what I mean by simulation being a technology of affect: it produces and modifies affect through expert knowledge structures (i.e., professionalism) in order to make up certain types of people (here, the professional physician who embodies the medical habitus). However, simulation is fraught with an interesting tension between authenticity and artificiality that must be managed if it is to be successful. The success of simulation thus hinges on its affective resonance. In this way, affect is central to these subject-making practices.

Authenticity and Artificiality in Simulation

In the medical schools from which I recruited, the students first try out their exam skills on a plastic model before seeing the GTA. These models vary in quality and sophistication, as well as age. Medical faculty reported that practicing on these models was useful for students to learn the basic techniques, but that to truly learn students had to examine an actual person. As MD medical faculty member Sakura explained:

> The [important thing] is being able to do these exams on an actual person. . . . The models cannot simulate what an actual body is like. And even our models . . . we got some brand new ones, they're very good, they're very expensive, but they . . . are not the same as a human body. . . . It's just not possible with plastic to simulate the pliability and elasticity of human tissue. And just the way that human tissue responds to pressure. That . . . can't be simulated using plastic.

What makes examining a real person valuable, then, is that biomedical technology so far does not have a type of plastic model that accurately simulates the experience of performing a pelvic exam on a living person. Living tissue palpates differently than synthetic tissue in simulation models or the decaying tissue found in a cadaver. When ethical dilemmas about using clinic patients were first considered among medical educators in the 1960s and 1970s, cadavers were posited as a possible solution to this dilemma (Beckmann et al. 1988; Kapsalis 1997). However, a living person is essential. As medical student Basil explained:

With the cadaver, a lot of those organs are withered away. And those relationships . . . aren't preserved so well, specifically with the liga- ments and the arteries and stuff like that. . . . You can read as much as you want about these maneuvers and manipulations, but until you're doing it . . . sweeping across the pelvis, feeling for ovaries, until you do that, do you realize, oh wait a second, all those ligaments are actually not fixed. . . . They move and here I am moving them and I can feel the texture of the ovaries.

I spoke of the shift from the cadaver to the GTA and simulated patient in the introduction. In Basil's explanation, this shift becomes central. Even rehearsing the exam skills on a cadaver is not adequate for medical students to obtain a suitable understanding of how the anatomy should feel during the exam. In addition, performing a pelvic exam on a GTA involves more than getting the feel of living tissue, given that a GTA can provide feedback. A GTA is not merely a living body who passively allows the pelvic exam to be performed; a GTA is a living *person* animated by affect.

Even as inexperienced as they are, medical students understand this. For example, medical student Ted said: "I think the models help with the basic stuff, but it is almost totally different. It's different from a real person. I mean, some of the things they are showing are very subtle." While the medical students I interviewed felt, in general, as though the plastic models were useful for reducing their anxiety about the actual mechanics of the exam, they also understood and could readily feel the difference between plastic and living human tissue. Thus, in order to gain appreciation for how actual tissue feels, medical students need the experience of actually touching living tissue. This demonstrates the im- portant role of the embodied development of perception as part of the medical habitus. To learn how to accurately *feel* through the technique of physical palpation, medical students depend on the physical sensa- tions of their bodies and the ways in which their own bodies move dur- ing the exam.

However, the pelvic exam involves more than manual-technical skills, as I have said. A physician must also interact with a sensate person in a competent and caring way. What simulation encounters like GTAs do is allow medical students an opportunity to rehearse both the manual skills and the piece of the exam that requires them to interact with real people. MD medical faculty member Elizabeth explained:

> You can't take a piece of plastic and put a speculum in it. It's not the same. . . . It's more than just . . . how do you use a speculum, how to attach the light, how to use a cytobrush, but it's about how do you talk to a female patient about what you're about to do, how do you approach the patient, how do you talk before touch. And so we need a lot of students to practice that so that when they are in an environment where they are doing that pelvic exam on an actual patient that they're able to reflect that on that experience that they had.

What came up in my interviews with medical faculty, students, and the coordinators of GTA programs is that there is no substitute for performing the exam on a living person who can talk back and who expects to be treated with a certain level of care and dignity. This is what the controversy at the University of Minnesota in 2010 demonstrates. Plastic models are helpful for learning the basic movements and techniques or "procedural skills," but to learn the subtleties of correct language and attitude and to learn how to appear confidence and competent, medical students must perform the exam on a real, sensate person, especially given the shift in clinical medicine from treating patients as inert bodies on whom physicians deploy their expertise to engaging them as active subjects who participate in their medical treatment.

While students may be nervous about forgetting steps or knowing normal from abnormal, I claim that what they are most nervous about is the *affect* of the encounter: appearing incompetent in front of the patient, being embarrassed or embarrassing the patient, hurting the patient. These moments of tension are about both the medical student and the patient's embodied experiences of emotion. With the pelvic exam in particular, the need for appropriate management of one's own and the patient's *affective disposition* is heightened, and students are more nervous about the potential for error. As medical student Michelle said:

> I think it has to do with the fact that on top of the invasive exam, you also have to connect with the person and maintain a rapport and interact with them just as you do anybody that you see on the street. . . . I guess

the presence of the sensitive exam sort of poses the question, "Oh, am I talking to them right?" . . . Which of course you don't have to worry about [with] the dummy. . . . You don't have to worry about [making] a dummy comfortable or putting them at ease.

Thus, what makes working with a GTA so important is that medical students need real people to learn how to navigate the affective components of the exam, the part where fleshy human beings—patient and physician—have feelings and emotional responses to what is physically happening.

However, medical students are cognizant of the artificiality of GTA sessions. While they appreciate performing the exam on a real, living person, they also are aware that the GTA session only simulates the experience of performing the pelvic exam on a clinic patient. Just as students appreciated the differences between plastic models and real bodies, they also noticed a difference between a GTA who is trained and comfortable and a clinic patient who most likely is not. Medical student Jeff said:

GTAs are healthy, normal [lacking pathology], and will give you feedback. Patients may not be healthy, may not be normal, don't really give you feedback. . . . They're all tensed up and they're scared, embarrassed, for whatever reason. Not all people are like that, but the [GTA] teacher is very comfortable, very inviting, engaging, because they're for teaching you.

But to take the point further, even as GTAs allow students to experience interacting with a human being, GTAs do not simulate being a nervous, scared, or embarrassed patient. Here, it would seem as though the correlation between the simulated environment and the real-world encounter breaks down (Hoffman 2006). However, medical faculty emphasize that while this is true, medical students neither have the experience nor do they need to experience a terrified, tense patient to learn from the encounter. As MD medical faculty member Miriam told me:

The students seem to find it useful to be able to practice things first. I think there is some variation. . . . Sometimes the students say, oh, this is not, you know, this doesn't feel real, it's not like the real patient. But the residents know, yes, this is like the real patient so sometimes the students because of their lack of experience don't realize it.

When I asked medical faculty about simulation, I heard time and again that rehearsal is what is most important. Medical students need to have a real body animated by affect if they are to become competent enough with any type of clinical skill to be able to safely perform it on a real patient. And, as I have shown, what makes the GTA session especially important is learning to deal with one's own and the patient's emotions. Affect cannot be simulated or reproduced by medical technologies, even as sophisticated as many are today.

The GTA experience is also noticeably artificial because of the difference in standards between it and the clinical setting. Medical students work with GTAs and other simulated patients during first- and second-year courses on basic patient interaction and exam skills, and the communication skills that the GTA program uses, such as "talk before touch" and neutral feedback, are emphasized in every unit of these courses. The medical students I interviewed expressed awareness that there is a distinct difference between what is expected to pass the test in the course and what happens in the clinical setting. Christopher explained:

> You know, they're [clinical encounters] rushed. So there's two sets of standards, basically. There's the [course] standard. . . . So, there's [course] language, [course] standards, and then the real world standards. . . . you can't say, I'm going to take a look, or I'm going to touch, or I'm going to feel [in the course]. . . . You have to say either inspect, check, or examine.

Other students similarly told stories about the differences between course standards and so-called real-world standards. Students went through the GTA session and learned the standardized language and skills, but then went into the clinic and watched their preceptors and faculty practice in a completely different way. The adherence to course principles such as "talk before touch" and using "ICE" words is not as strict in the actual clinic as it is in workshops. These differences are due to the corporatized nature of the US health system: the length of time physicians have with patients is shrinking while the amount of tasks they must complete is growing. As a result, some students even reported being chastised for attempting to maintain course standards in the clinic. In this way, medical students who came into the GTA encounter with some clinical experience were especially cognizant of the artificiality of the situation.

This artificiality was also noted by medical faculty who were concerned with students' ability to perform in actual clinical practice. Elizabeth told me that "you get people who think they're really good in a standardized setting and then you put them in an actual human being setting and they're not so good." Medical faculty admitted in my interviews that sometimes students performed the pelvic exam on GTAs very well and likewise demonstrated excellent interpersonal skills in that context, but when faced with an actual patient, became too nervous or uncertain to perform the exam. In an artificial context, the stakes aren't as high as the real-world clinic, so medical students may perform better in the simulation encounter. In this way, the quality of the affective experience is different in simulation than in the clinic.

Thus, the GTA encounter exists in a tenuous space between the performance of an authentic clinical encounter and the artificiality of a simulated encounter. As Hoffman argues, the "effectiveness of a simulation thus depends on . . . how well participants translate the imperfect fit between contextual norms of the simulation and the reality it is based on" (2006:172). Standards may be different from the clinical encounter, GTAs may not totally act like real patients, and techniques that may work on one GTA may not work on every person. Yet the GTA session remains effective, though it is noticeably artificial, because medical students are able to translate the encounter from simulation to clinic through its affective resonance. This highlights the crucial role of the affective labor performed by GTAs.

Affective Resonance and Intimate Labor in Simulation

To engage in simulation requires agreement between medical students and the "fake patients" that they practice on about what is and isn't authentic or real. To make something *feel* real, however, to make the simulation feel as though it matches the real world, requires work. *Because GTAs make the encounter safe, comfortable, and nonthreatening, while* at the same time allowing medical students to practice the emotional dispositions of medical culture, this simulation works to begin the process of professional socialization. In this way, the inculcation of the medical habitus in medical students depends in part on the intimate labor that GTAs perform.

GTAs attempt to create an emotionally resonant simulation of the human interaction of performing a pelvic exam. They attempt to be as authentic as possible so that medical students can have the experience of examining real people, with their range of emotions, elastic tissue, and potential sexuality (but not, as I discuss in chapter 1, their menstrual fluids). However, GTAs cannot act like clinic patients, and nor do they *want* to, for all of the reasons I discuss in chapter 3: they have to protect their bodies from harm and from unwanted intimacy, even as they are working to support medical students' educational experience. Their intimate labor is bounded: they "sell" genuine patient encounters without themselves being genuine patients, with all the emotional and physical vulnerability that that entails.[9]

Lena, a coordinator, emphasized many times that she trains and hires her GTAs with an emphasis on the student experience: "We're there because we want to improve healthcare . . . but I also think we're there for the students. . . . I want there to be better healthcare for the patient, but also an important learning activity for the students, to support them and help them learn." When Lena first took over managing several programs, there was resistance to her emphasis on teaching students first and getting "the politics out of the exam room." Lena emphasizes giving students the opportunity to practice their communication and manual exam techniques in a safe, supportive environment. In describing the type of person she likes to hire as a GTA, Lena said:

> I like people who . . . physically aren't going to be intimidating. . . . I like people who have a nice . . . supportive demeanor. Somebody who comes prepared, really knows their stuff, so I do like smart people. . . . And the supporting, and the smart thing, to me they just kind of go hand in hand because . . . sometimes it would honestly get a little bit argumentative between the teachers and the students. . . . We have to learn how to work with them because . . . if you think they're being snippy, the student might

be snippy for a number of different reasons and . . . I think we need to try
to support them rather than put it to them or whatever.

This is in sharp contrast to some of the early feminist politics that
I discussed in chapter 1. Lena's GTAs are there to attend to the student experience in order to improve healthcare for patients. Thus, the
low-risk environment of simulation is produced actively through the
intimate labor of the GTA. It is not merely that she is not a real patient,
but that she is constantly managing her emotion to support the student.

Lena wasn't the only program coordinator who wanted supportive
GTAs to teach the pelvic exam. Other coordinators and medical faculty also emphasized the importance of someone who is knowledgeable
about the anatomy and the clinical skills but who is also supportive and
a good teacher. As program coordinator Heather explained:

> I think there's a really strong importance to patient instructors [like
> GTAs]. . . . They've experienced working with the students a lot year after
> year, so they kind of know the right balance of things, how they come
> to answer their question, how to make them comfortable, *how not to
> scare them too much.* But how to just make it simple and clear. (Emphasis
> added.)

It bears mentioning that GTAs perform this intimate labor of being nice
and supportive to students while simultaneously receiving an invasive
physical exam. There is the potential for physical harm for GTAs, which
is why they need techniques to control the encounter. And yet, GTAs try
not to react or express too much discomfort if a student makes a mistake
lest it frighten the student.

The importance and gendered nature of GTAs' intimate labor is evident in the kinds of responses medical students gave when I asked their
impressions of the GTA they worked with. Almost all of them talked
about how comfortable the GTAs made them feel. Amber explained to
me that "they put an enormous part into making you feel comfortable."
GTAs were "helpful," "nice," "friendly," and put the students at ease.
Roger said that GTAS "end up being someone you can sort of trust and
feel comfortable with." This type of intimate labor is what Kapsalis (1997)

criticized in her account of working as a GTA in Chicago-area medical schools during the late 1980s and 1990s. She argued that that the GTA is like a flight attendant in that "she is there to make the student's trip through the female body comfortable, safe and enjoyable" (1997:77). Thus, while medical students need to practice on real bodies inhabited by the sociality of their patients, the sociality of the GTA is not necessarily the goal. She is *playing* herself, but she cannot *be* herself. She has to learn when and how to deploy her sociality in the teaching encounter to support the students.

The intimate labor performed by GTAs serves to make an artificial encounter feel more authentic, and it allows GTAs to provide a low-risk environment for medical students to learn to conduct an emotionally fraught exam in a competent, patient-friendly manner. The skills associated with emotion management that medical student learn are two-fold and highlight the intersubjective nature of affect: at the same time that students learn to manage their own emotions, they learn to manage the emotions of the patient. Thus, GTAs help prepare medical students to engage in the kind of affective discipline that will be required of them in the clinical setting.

Performing Emotion in Clinical Practice

Thus far this chapter has explored how the GTA session helps shape the subjectivities of medical students. I now turn to the values and norms that are evident in medical training under this contemporary regime of affect and have important implications for the kind of clinical practice that students are being prepared to undertake. As my colleagues and I have shown, emotional labor has become central to clinical practice (Underman and Hirshfield 2016; Vinson and Underman 2020). Likewise, in an article in the *Journal of the American Medical Association*, health professions scholars Eric B. Larson and Xin Yao write: "In the patient-physician relationship, social behaviors such as communication and a considerate social style (e.g., warmth, sensitivity, positive outlook, and even temper) are the main concern" (2005:1102). Further: "We take a psychological approach and define emotional labor as the process of regulating experienced and displayed emotions to present a professionally desired image during interpersonal transactions at work" (Larson and Yao 2005:1103). Teaching acting skills to physicians, they argue, will allow physicians to both "activate empathic processes" and "help them achieve detachment when they become too engaged in a patient's experience" (Larson and Yao 2005:1105). As of 2019, this article had been cited almost 800 times, and the range of citations indicate the radical shift from detached concern to "clinical empathy" in medical education.

I argue that a *routinized performance of empathy* is increasingly important to clinical practice under the contemporary regime of affect in medical education. Empathy as a teachable skillset has emerged from medical education research and serves to discipline the conduct of physicians as they in turn shape the conduct of their patients. The communication skills that medical students learn in the GTA session are generally in line with those they learn in other simulated encounters. In the three medical schools I studied, the GTA session occurs as a unit in an ongoing course in professionalism. Skills such as "talk before touch," using "ICE words," or displaying compassion and empathy are taught throughout these courses. At one of the schools I studied, students are given an index-card sized "cheat sheet" that breaks down skills associated with empathy to keep in the pocket of their whitecoats. Simulated patients are likewise trained to teach and evaluate skills associated with empathy in trainees—even in national licensing exams. As many recent studies show, however, assessing empathy is incredibly challenging.[10]

Medical students rarely spoke of these difficulties.[11] However, I did have an informative exchange with Christopher, which was later echoed in informal conversations with medical students and in the literature. Christopher was generally positive about the GTA encounter, but when it came to its broader context—the professionalism course—he became quickly critical. Specifically, his criticisms were about the evaluation side.

> They're very uptight about the finesse part of seeing patient. . . . You have to watch every word that you say with them. . . . In my introduction to the pelvic exam, I was saying, okay, I'm checking the skin and the hair here for any lesions, and she [the GTA] cut me off, she said, Oh, no, no, don't say lesions. That might make the patient worry. So it's a huge contrast between the workshops and the actual clinic . . . the attendings don't have these high standards.

The gap between the standards in a simulated encounter and those in a clinical session has also been noted by sociologists. Indeed, this is what the legacy of the hidden curriculum perspective gives us (Hafferty and Castellani 2009). Medical students are taught one thing in their formal curriculum and another thing by their attendings in the clinic, a space in which medical hierarchies dominate. This disconnect is indeed quite revealing about the challenges of training medical students to adopt this routinized performance of empathy. The emphasis on standardization and scientific ways of teaching and learning about emotion bumps up against the structural constraints of clinical practice, as I argue in chapter 2. These gaps and fissures are exposed, in part, in the ways in which medical students grapple with actually performing emotion in the clinic. I return to this theme in the conclusion.

The challenge of standardizing teaching and learning empathy is no small problem, and not limited solely to a couple of courses that medical students take. This challenge is only going to increase, as institutionalized controls reward physicians who can conform to the performance of empathy appropriately and sanction those who do not. The inclusion in 2012 of questions about managing patient emotion on the USMLE is but one example. Another is that physicians are incentivized by insurance companies to get high scores on patient satisfaction measures. With the rise of websites like Yelp and HealthGrades allowing patients to publicly share experiences they have had with their physicians, the corporatized orientation of the profession increasingly begins to depend on catering to the emotional needs of patients. Thus, I am not optimistic about the incorporation of emotional labor into clinical practice—or about clinical empathy more broadly. I am interested instead in the ways in which learning to manage patient emotions becomes a tool for the continued maintenance of the professional dominance of medicine. This is affective governance at work.

5

"What Does It Mean to Relax Your Hand?"

Learning to Feel with the Body in the Pelvic Exam

Simulation is a practice that demonstrates the drive toward standardization in medical education. Using simulated patients is intended to ensure that all medical students learn the same skills and can be evaluated on these on more or less equal basis, as explored in the previous chapters. And yet, as I argue throughout this book, the practice of medicine in the clinic is thoroughly saturated with affect. Attending to bodily capacities to affect and be affected by the material world remains a crucial piece of the work of being a physician, even as a proliferation of diagnostic technologies render the patient's body into a collection of *dis*embodied points of data. Consider, for example, the following passage:

> The cervix is felt with two fingers of the left hand in the vagina. Note the location and consistency of the cervix. An especially soft cervix . . . or an especially hard cervix . . . should both be noted. Then place the right hand on the patient's lower abdomen. . . . The uterus is usually palpated as a pear-shaped organ. . . . It may be lifted with the vaginal fingers for greater ease of palpation. Ordinarily it is firm, smooth, movable, and nontender. Notations should be made of any abnormality in its size, shape, symmetry, consistency, or mobility. (Long 1990:828)

This description of conducting a bimanual examination, which comes from a medical textbook, *Clinical Methods: The History, Physical, and Laboratory Methods*, is intended to prepare medical students for how the reproductive anatomy should feel. And yet, this passage is quite opaque with regard to sensation. Certainly, feeling matters. The cervix *is felt* and what is felt matters diagnostically (a soft cervix could mean pregnancy while a hard cervix could mean cancer). The uterus *is felt*. In fact, it is lifted and felt, and information is taken from this lifting and feeling of the uterus (an enlarged uterus in a nonpregnant patient could mean fibroids).

Can you imagine what the anatomy would feel like by reading this passage? Does calling the uterus "pear-shaped" help you understand the sensations in your hands when cupping it between them? If you have palpated a uterus before, perhaps this conjures some bodily memories. But for those who have not, the passage likely seems abstract. And it is—this description elides all of the tacit knowledge about feeling that is crucial for performing the pelvic exam. Sensation matters here and is part of the work of the pelvic exam, but sensation cannot be translated through written (or even spoken) language. In this way, sensation is a remainder, affect a residual category (Guarrasi 2015). The expert attends to it in dynamic, non-articulated ways. Therefore, for medical students to become experts, they too must learn how to attend to sensation in a manner specific to the clinic.[1]

In this chapter, I argue that GTAs train medical students to become attuned to the sensations in the students' own bodies in order to examine the body of another. This process is particularly interesting in the context of teaching and learning the pelvic exam. The objects of the medical students' attention—cervix, ovaries, and uterus—are enclosed within the body of another person, and learning to discern organs, healthy or diseased, relies on learning to "read" one's own bodily sensations appropriately. In my case, this other person is simultaneously relying upon haptic knowledge to teach the exam. This educational process creates novel tensions and troubles thinking of the body in terms of subjects and objects, insides and outsides, parts and wholes. I offer this analysis to illustrate some of the difficulties of theorizing the body in medicine. The body is *constructed* in practice—the uterus must be felt and must be described as firm, smooth, and movable, marking it as *normal*. But the uterus that is felt exists prior to the exam, in which medical knowledge is applied to it, and it acts on the physician's hand by producing these sensations. Thus, by posing the question of how medical students learn to feel in the GTA session, I argue that feeling is a collectivized, embodied practice, in which affects circulate within and between bodies, in culturally specific ways. I call this learning to "feel with," a concept I develop here to attend to the perceptual, embodied, and affective dimensions of clinical practice.

"Feeling with" as Clinical Perception

Learning to feel with the body in the pelvic exam is a process by which medical trainees become attuned to the sensations of their own bodies in order to make *objects of knowledge* out of the interior spaces of another person's body. This involves the use of material objects such as specula and gloves, which affect the how a trainee registers sensation. I develop this notion of *feeling with* to challenge some of the existing literature on medical embodiment, which largely ignores sensation and, moreover, presumes that physicians and patients inhabit separate, self-contained bodies.[2] "Feeling with" attends to the ways in which physicians' and patients' bodies co-produce one another in the clinical encounter and are likewise co-produced by medical discourse. Furthermore, I develop this concept to understand the limits of standardization in medical work. Sensation—as the capacity of bodies to register movement and difference in the world—is inherently incapable of being captured by standardizing technologies, and learning to grapple with it accordingly is a key aspect of professional socialization in medical education.

Central to my development of "feeling with" is the role of perception. I call it *clinical perception* to capture the unique forms of medical embodiment that arise out of training for and practicing in the clinical setting. In general, *perception* is the production and awareness of differences out of a constant and always already occurring flow of experience. Another way to think of perception is as a material engagement with the world that provides the subject with knowledge. Thus, "feeling with" is a mode of clinical perception that encompasses the body of the trainee or physician, the body of the patient, and all of the material objects in the clinical space. I draw from phenomenological and new materialist accounts of perception to understand medical embodiment in this way.

Phenomenological accounts describe the body as not merely an object among objects, but as the vehicle through which we experience the world.[3] We create objects by focusing our attention on them *as objects* (meaning, as distinct from our own sense of where our bodies begin and end). Knowledge about the world occurs as perception, as a cohesive link between our minds and bodies as we move through the world. This way of theorizing the body and knowledge allows phenomenologists to overcome the subject/object binary. For example, philosopher Maurice Merleau-Ponty (2013) provides the example of a blind person navigating a room with a cane. Held tightly and used to navigate, the cane is an extension of the body that enhances the person's ability to perceive the surrounding world. Held loosely and used, perhaps, to lean on, the cane is an object distinct from the body. Perception, thus, is about registering differences in a constantly varying and changing realm of experience. In this way, perception can be of the world around us or of our own internal worlds. This tangles up the positionality of the knower and the known, just as it tangles up subject and object. Touch is one of the primary modes of perception that mixes up insides and outsides of bodies, especially self-touch, since we feel through our hand even as our hand feels our elbow or knee or whatever body part we are touching (Barad 2012; Harris 2016).

This work on perception incorporates new materialist perspectives on sensation as an embodied registering of affect. Brian Massumi (2002) theorizes that affect is a sort of intensity that is lived at the level of the body and exists prior to thought, language, and awareness. Affect is two-sided: it is both a realm of pure potentiality, wherein the body relates only to its own ability to move and act in the world, and it is the body's registering of these differences in systems of signification or discourse (Massumi 2002).[4] These two sides of affect collide through movement, in the body's "immediate, unfolding relation to its own . . . potential to vary" (Massumi 2002:4). Just as in phenomenology, the body knows and experiences simultaneously, in affect theory, the body registers and moves simultaneously. Sensation is thus an *effect* of affect; it is a registering in the body of the immanence and intensities of experience. Sensation is central to perception, since it produces the difference for the body to note.

In the clinic, sensation plays an important role in making bodies. The bodies of medical trainees are crafted in distinct ways as they engage in more and more clinical practices such as inspection, palpation, percussion, and auscultation[5] (Harris 2016; Prentice 2013). The trainee's body opens up to novel worlds of sensation and movement that are inseparable from the production of knowledge in the clinical encounter. Writing on medical trainees learning self-percussion, anthropologist Anna Harris argues that in doing so [learning to self-percuss], the materiality of bodies comes to the fore, dissolving boundaries between the perceiver and the perceived, the skilled expert and the object of learning, highlighting how perception is not only of something external to the self, but can also be internal and inextricably tied up with the cultivation of one's own body and other bodies. Perception is not, or not always, a registration of some world out there by means of separated sensory organs, but rather an intricate engagement in which knower and known are crafted together, through sensing in movement. (2016:23)

Likewise, Gili Hammer argues that the process of attending to sensation "opens avenues between external and internal sensations, between teachers' and students' bodies, and between the 'knower'—the student/medical novice—and the 'known'—the information being given in class (a body part or a bone, a treatment method, a diagnostic practice, a specific pathology)" (2018:148). In this way, bodies become alive to new modes of being that are intrinsic to clinical knowledge-making.

New modes of clinical perception rely upon the materiality of the trainee's own body, the patient's body, and the material objects in the clinical space. In this way, "feeling with" relies upon new materialist accounts that theorize matter as co-productive of or entangled with agencies of perception. In her path-breaking book *Meeting the Universe Halfway*, physicist and feminist philosopher Karen Barad (2007) argues that discourse and materiality are *intra*-active (as opposed to *inter*active), meaning that matter and meaning are always already co-constitutive. Discourse acts on matter, even as matter "kicks back" onto discourse, causing one to shape the other.[6] In her work on intra-action, boundaries between subjects and objects are constructed through specific discursive practices. Measurement is one kind of discursive practice that produces what is subject and what is object.[7] Here Barad is drawing from phenomenology, wherein the object comes into being by being focused upon *as an object*, but she is critical of the centrality of the subject. Because matter and meaning are *intra*-active, knowledge and world-making are inseparable. To know the body is to enact the material, and vice versa.

Thus, knowing and being are inseparable, and in this way, learning to "feel with" is a mode of being and knowing the material world produced by and through the assemblage of the pelvic exam, which requires the embodied presences of both physician and patient. In processes of feeling with, a body learns how to experience its own affective capacities in relationship to the affective capacities of other bodies (human and nonhuman); it becomes attuned to novel sensations and learns to register different types of sensations in order to produce information in culturally specific ways. By learning to feel with their own bodies, medical students tangle up inside and outside as they make knowledge about the material world (here, the patient). Again, my conceptualization of "feeling with" therefore points to the limits of science and standardization in medicine, since attending to constant variation in the material world is a key piece of clinical work.

Learning to "Feel with" the Body in the Pelvic Exam

Throughout their training, medical students are taught how to "see" like a physician or adopt the medical gaze: they are taught physiology, anatomy, and biology, so that they can thoroughly understand the human body as the object of their knowledge. And yet, this does not mean that bodies are always objects or that medical students always ignore the patient's inner life.[8] Far from it, in fact. What it means is that there are long-standing and deeply embedded tensions in clinical practice between modes of knowing, between the body as a known object from the outside and the body as felt from within (Mol and Law 2004). For medical students to become expert physicians—for them to really know the body that they are examining—they must engage with it materially at the same time as they become attuned to their own bodies. This is the first and most embodied sense of what I mean by "feeling with": medical students must be made to attend to their bodily sensations in order to fully learn the pelvic exam.

This is apparent in my interviews with medical students as they describe the process of learning the pelvic exam. As with all aspects of clinical practice, learning to perform the pelvic exam begins with a large amount of scientific, technical, and anatomical knowledge that is abstracted from bodily experience. In my interviews, I asked medical students how they were prepared to go into the GTA session. While specifics vary by school, in general medical students have a large number of materials about pelvic anatomy and pathology to learn before they perform the exam on the GTA. Medical students typically study a textbook such as *A Clinical Manual of Gynecology*, attend a lecture by a faculty member, watch a video, and read materials explaining the exam from the patient's point of view, such as an article by a woman physician, who describes the feelings of helplessness and shame that accompany being examined in this way (Magee 1975). However, the bulk of the emphasis is on learning the anatomy so that medical students can go into the session and apply it to the body of the patient. This knowledge, though, is inadequate, and the materials give very little information about how the exam itself is actually *felt* by the medical student.

Medical students told me repeatedly that their anatomical knowledge of the pelvis was either insufficient or didn't solidify until they practiced the exam on the GTA. Medical student Basil explained:

> In all honesty, I was as nervous as ever because I've never done anything like that in . . . the clinical setting. So I knew the anatomy and I memorized the phrases everybody was supposed to say and whatnot, but none of that really matters when you're in front of the patient and . . . you're actually expected to perform.

He then went on to say:

> You know the general layout of pelvic anatomy, and you can tell the story of how it developed and whatnot, but . . . the physical relationships that . . . are so important for surgical and clinical manipulation . . . you can't appreciate any of that . . . from a textbook. . . . You can just feel, here are the sizes, here are the appropriate textures, the appropriate pressure points. And, I mean for me, that's when everything kind of clicked.

For Basil and other medical students who answered similarly, anatomical knowledge of the pelvis can take a medical student only so far in knowing how to perform the pelvic exam and understanding pelvic anatomy. It isn't until medical students perform the exam that the knowledge "clicks." Knowing the body requires the medical student to engage materially in practice with it, to attend to the sensations that another body evokes. In this way, medical knowledge of the body arises from the embodied perception of the medical student or experienced physician. Medical students must learn to feel with their own bodies.

Similarly, medical student Daphne told me about the videos her class had to watch, noting that "it's a lot harder to translate—it's kind of like trying to learn how to dance by just watching a video. . . . It's much easier . . . practicing it on a model or a person than reading it in a book." Daphne's language here evokes some of Massumi's discussion of proprioception: dancers needs the feel of the floor against their feet and the feeling of their bodies moving in space to know how to dance. Likewise, Kathleen told me that "you can see diagrams of that [anatomy] but until you feel . . . it, it's really just imagination." Thus, the medical gaze may mean that "the gaze that sees is the gaze that dominates" (Foucault 1994), but knowing the body from the outside as an object is only one mode of knowing. The clinical encounter requires modes of knowing that merge objective and subjective forms of knowledge. However, learning the body in the pelvic exam is unlike other ways of knowing the body, as my discussion of Marie's experience of teaching the pelvic exam to her friend's partner in chapter 3 illustrates. Knowing the body in a sexual relationship or friendship may involve the same body parts, but the context is entirely different. Medical students must become alive to sensation in novel and clinically specific ways.

Medical student Roger described the process of learning the pelvic exam in a way that highlights the importance of the sensorial relationship between the medical student and the object of knowledge as well as the affects that circulate in the exam:

> Seeing it and doing it are two different things. You can see someone and they are like, "Yes, do you see what I am doing?" and you are like "Yeah, I see what you are doing," but do you know exactly where to put your hands, what kind of pressure to use and things like that? You also don't know what the patient experience is going to be like . . . so it's a chance to sort of judge a patient's reaction and the chance to sort of refine your . . . skills, make sure that you are putting your hands in the right place and doing the right things.

Here, Roger again highlights the importance of literally getting his hands on the body of the patient in order to fully understand the exam.

However, Roger takes this a step further and adds the patient's affect into the thing to be experienced: he had to learn to "judge a patient's reaction" on top of learning all of the technical skills. His ability to learn to feel with depended on a mode of attention that included both his own embodiment *and* the embodied presence of another.

GTAs likewise emphasized the importance of students being encouraged to focus on sensation as part of the learning process. For example, Sylvia said:

> You could tell the students felt more comfortable when the patient was engaging in teaching them . . . whereas if somebody else is standing there and they're turning to them, saying, "Is this right?" [*Laughs*] They're not learning to check in with the patient, say, "Does this feel uncomfortable? Let me know if this feels uncomfortable." They're not learning those skills. They're [not] learning . . . to count on their own tactile senses. More to rely on somebody else outside . . . of the patient who's in the best position to give them that kind of information.

Sylvia and other GTAs who shared her view emphasize that the importance of this model of teaching is to get students to start learning to count on their own senses and to interact with the patient's experience of the exam. What all of this demonstrates is that learning is embodied: medical students cannot fully understand or appreciate the anatomical information that they are acquiring without literally getting their hands on it—without being able to practice on a living person and experience those anatomical relationships for themselves. In another sense, learning is embodied in that it requires the presence of two bodies: the medical student's and the patient's. Developing one's own embodied perception is tied to the knowledge about the material world (i.e., the patient's body) that one is acquiring. As I will underscore throughout this chapter, this has important implications for what it means to be an expert: one's expertise cannot be separated from one's embodiment.

"Feeling with" and Intra-Active Modes of Attention

Becoming alive to their own bodily sensations is important in order for medical students to develop the skills necessary to do the pelvic exam—and to truly acquire the knowledge of the human body. But how do medical students learn to make their objects of knowledge? By this I mean how are subjects and objects created through practice or "enacted" (Mol and Law 2004) by shifts in embodied perception? How does this occur between as well as within bodies? How are bodily exteriors enacted and how are objects within bodies enacted by shifting modes of attention? These questions are highly relevant for the pedagogical work done by GTAs. Their work exemplifies the inseparability of being and knowing, and they use embodied perception to teach in ways that makes it difficult to distinguish when they're subject and when they're object or what parts of them are which at any given moment. In this way, learning to feel with is an intra-active mode of attention, in that it endlessly shifts the boundaries between subject and object.

As I described in chapter 3, the GTAs I interviewed expressed their knowledge of their own bodies and bodily sensations with a high level of detail. A typical GTA is able to tell from bodily sensation whether the proper organs are being palpated, the placement of the speculum, and so forth. GTAs develop this knowledge over the course of many experiences receiving the pelvic exam. The GTAs and the program coordinators whom I interviewed all stressed the importance of a training process that combined teaching anatomy and pathology with practicing the exam itself. Lena is the program coordinator and owner of a company in Chicago that contracts out GTAs, genitor-urinary teaching associates for the prostate exam, and standardized patients to all of the major medical schools. In Lena's program, GTAs both experience the exam on their own bodies and have to practice the exam on each other in order to be considered fully trained. As they do in other programs in Chicago, GTAs go through multiple sessions learning how it feels to have a proper exam before they are able to teach. Training involves learning to pair specific sensations with particular biomedical techniques, which a typical layperson would encounter only once a year at most during a clinical exam. Over the course of weeks and years of experience, GTAs can tell by the bodily sensations that they have learned to identify whether students' technique is correct.

GTAs' knowledge of the material world is thus inseparable from their embodied state of being. Knowledge about their own bodies, the bodies of their students, and the tools and instruments involved in the

pelvic exam cannot exist without attunement to sensation and movement. GTAs make objects of knowledge by focusing their attention on
them and training medical students to do the same. This is what I mean
by learning to feel with the body. In this way, the pedagogical work of
GTAs mixes up existing bodily boundaries. Or, to put this a slightly different way, the practice of the pelvic exam makes objects out of wholes
and parts for both patient and physician. This being and knowing arise
from configurations of materiality and discourse specific to the pelvic
exam.[9]

For example, medical students often have a difficult time identifying ovaries. It is a persistent problem in the pelvic exam at any level of
medical practice, as ovaries are very small and not fixed in the pelvis the
way that the uterus is. Even though it can be considered normal to not
palpate the ovaries (meaning, find and assess for size, texture, and so
forth) during a regular exam, it is an important part of the GTA session
since medical students are unlikely to have a trained and willing person
to practice on again. In addition, the logic is that students should have
some experience knowing what normal is so that they can more readily
identify abnormal. Therefore, GTAs have to learn to identify a particular
twinge or sensation and link it to being produced by palpating the ovary
so that they can clue medical students in to the technique. Program coordinator Donna describes this training process:

> You had to figure out like, oh, that's my cervix, okay, yeah I can feel
> that. You had to be able to recognize when your ovary was being palpated
> so you could tell the student, oh, I just felt that, did you feel that? ... And
> be able to give them specific feedback about their manual skills.

Prior to the recognition that that particular twinge is an ovary or a cervix being palpated, these organs do not exist as objects of knowledge
for the medical student or GTA. Through the GTA learning to register
these novel sensations, the ovary or cervix becomes an object of knowledge. Its existence as an object of knowledge holds together only so long
as this enactment occurs in the pelvic exam. Outside of this particular
material-discursive practice, ovaries and cervixes are different kinds
of objects, if they are objects at all.[10] Accordingly, as Donna's description illustrates, this pedagogical work entails the GTA feeling with the

medical student in this intra-active fashion ("I just felt that, did you feel that?").

Consider, for example, teaching speculum insertion. During insertion of the speculum, it can be very easy for a novice to "miss" the cervix and assume that a portion of the vaginal wall is the cervix. The tissue all looks quite similar, shiny and pink, and textbook descriptions or observation of a video or skilled practitioner can make it seem as though merely inserting the speculum is enough to get the cervix into view. In reality, cervices are small and can be finicky. Medical student Kathleen explains: "When I did the speculum [exam], one lady was like, okay . . . my cervix is it more in the middle. . . . Some days it's here and some days it's there." As medical student Ellie describes:

> [GTAs] can feel . . . how far your speculum is inserted during an exam into the vaginal canal. And they'll be able to tell you adjust that in or out so you get to the right spot where they think in their experience you'll be able to perform the exam better . . . to . . . observe the cervix . . . because it's on their body, and they can sort of sense these sorts of things. The communication from them is a valuable teaching tool in terms of kind of doing the exam properly.

Compare these descriptions to how GTA Grace explains teaching the speculum exam:

> I walk the first person through . . . and . . . explain to them how to press it [the speculum] in. . . . You want to rotate and press in until you feel pressure and then let it go just a little bit. Relieve your hand just a little bit because it doesn't have to be pushed in all the way on me. So just see where my body pressure pushes it out to and then open [it].

GTAs teach medical students to "read" their own bodies in order to adjust the speculum appropriately. During the speculum insertion, GTAs draw medical students' attention to the amount of downward pressure they're exerting on the speculum and the various feelings of resistance. When resistance becomes "bounce back," for example, the student knows they've inserted the speculum far enough. Or when the student is removing the speculum, there is a particular feeling of suction and then release that indicates that the cervix is no longer stuck on the lower bill.

Speculum insertion demonstrates the very complicated relationship among the objects of knowledge and "agencies of observation" (Barad 2007) that occur in the GTA session. GTAs tie particular sensations alive in movement to the practices of the pelvic exam and are able to render these objects of knowledge into pedagogical tools for medical students. At the same time, medical students likewise learn to attach meaning to their own bodily sensations. The GTA feels the speculum inside the vaginal canal and enacts the cervix as an object of knowledge. The medical student feels the motion of the speculum while inserting it into the vaginal canal and pairs that sensation with the technique. Only through doing this together can GTAs and medical students collectively make the cervix an object of medical knowledge. In this way, GTAs and medical students feel with one another and with the objects of their knowledge.

Thinking of feeling with as an intra-active mode of perception also allows me to draw on theories of the agency of materiality, which cast agency as the capacity of both human and nonhuman elements to act on other people and objects in the world (Barad 2007). One example of the agency of materiality is how the cervix moves around inside the GTA's body throughout the menstrual cycle, affecting the ways in which both the GTA and the medical student must learn to perceive it. This makes insertion of the speculum slightly more challenging, as GTAs must adjust their instruction in the moment based on feel and what the medical student sees in the speculum. Not only that, but the very type of speculum used complicates this. As Grace explains,

I must have four metal ones [specula] plus one plastic one [when I teach]. And I explain . . . what size I use and why, and the fact that when I first started, I started using medium. . . . Sometimes we'd see my cervix and sometimes we didn't. Then I used a large for a little while. We never saw my cervix. And now I use a small and we almost always see my cervix.

GTAs teach differently based on whether the speculum is plastic or metal, and whether or not they have access to the specific size of speculum that works best for their bodies on a given day.[11] Part of GTAs' work thus is helping medical students understand how their own bodily sensations will change depending on the tools available to them in a given clinical setting. In this way, feeling with as intra-active perception equips medical students with the ability to improvise in the moment, which all experts in clinical medicine have mastered.

For example, Marie describes how she teaches the bimanual exam to emphasize contingency and movement:

> Maybe someone is doing a bimanual exam and they can't find the cervix. . . . Their fingers are too short, or my arm's not long enough, I'm too short, or my leg is whatever, the table's bad. . . . I'm going to try my hardest to have them find the cervix and I'm going to explain to them many different ways to find the cervix.

Marie describes here common issues with the bimanual exam that emphasize the agency of materiality, both as parts of the body and tools of the clinic. Bodies are of course nonstandard: GTAs' bodies are "healthy and normal" in that they have intact uterus, cervix, and ovaries, but everything else about them varies, from whether their uterus is tipped forward or backward (anteverted or retroverted), to where their cervix is in their menstrual cycle. Likewise, the medical student's body is nonstandard. Students have different finger lengths, which affects how they're able to perform the exam: short fingers can make it difficult to reach the cervix. GTAs teach improvisation techniques that work with the student's body and sometimes the objects in the room, as when they recommend that the student prop a foot up on a stool and support the elbow on the knee to get better leverage. Feeling with acknowledges that bodies and objects differ, and it relies upon sensation and movement to provide workarounds.

Ruth likewise highlights this process:

> I have a pretty wily cervix, you know. I'm retroverted, retroflexed, so I have this cervix that kind of swims [laughs] . . . I'll give them [the students] specific instructions. . . . They need to tilt the speculum a certain way and rotate it a certain way and they'll find it nine times out of ten. But inevitably the question comes up, well, what if I don't find the cervix? . . . And I said, okay . . . we'll do it exactly the way the textbook tells us to insert the speculum and then we'll strategize. . . . And of course,

they don't find the cervix. So then I'll ask them, okay, so you can't find the cervix. Now let's just see. What do you think you should do? . . . They'll all say, okay, we'll add more posterior pressure and see what happens.

In Ruth's evocative discussion, medical students must learn to feel with their own bodies through the application of posterior pressure (pushing down on the speculum) in order to locate Ruth's cervix. She gives students the opportunity to practice the standard way, "the way the textbook tells us," and then she encourages them to rely on their instincts, knowledge, and—more importantly—their own bodily sensation in order to properly insert the speculum. This kind of variability of the GTA's body is welcomed by students as an opportunity to practice these workarounds. Tolerating uncertainty—the goal of medical training—means adopting these embodied dispositions that allow a physician to adjust to the wide variety of patient bodies and clinical settings.[12]

The importance of attending to sensation in these enactments is apparent when nonhuman bodies are introduced to teaching and learning the pelvic exam. Feeling with a nonhuman body is totally different. Many medical schools have adopted plastic or rubber models for medical students to practice their exam skills on (Epstein 2010). As I discussed in chapter 4, living tissue responds differently than the substance manikins are made of. In addition, manikins include only the reproductive organs, not any of the intestines, the bladder, or the adipose (fat) tissue that a medical student must examine around in order to find the reproductive organs that are the objects of knowledge for this particular exam. Some medical schools have adopted the use of haptic pelvic simulators, which are plastic models with inbuilt sensors to measure pressure. Often times, as I discuss in chapter 4, this is a response to budget cuts, as haptic simulators tend to be more cost-effective than GTAs in the long run.

However, there is a trade-off between cost and the style of practice that the medical student will develop. Haptic pelvic simulators emphasize the technical-manual skills of performing the pelvic exam, but do not allow for learning "the feel" of it. Anthropologist Rachel Prentice (2013) argues that such simulators abstract the technical from the experiential or subjective skill of clinical and surgical work and questions whether such technologies will result in a different form of practice. According to my interviews, they do. Medical faculty spoke of simulators as a first step to learn the technical-manual skill of the exam and to learn the gestures, hand positions, and locations of organs. None of the medical faculty viewed them as replacements for GTAs, though. GTAs themselves noticed that the practice tended to be different in medical students who had learned with haptic simulators. Vivian told me:

> They [the medical school] brought in these sort of like plastic models that had electronic gadgets that when the student touched the model ovary or the cervix, it would let them know . . . that the students would come in and work with those first and then they would come and do an exam. I noticed that what seemed to happen is that they would know more about . . . where to locate things, but they would press really hard because they had to get whatever the indicator was that they were in the right location.

A few other GTAs indicated similar aspects of the medical students' techniques when they initially worked with pelvic simulators. Medical students would press harder or would palpate in ways that were uncomfortable. The pelvic simulator is goal-oriented: find the cervix, the ovaries, and so forth. It doesn't have negative sensors, so to speak: nothing lights up or buzzes if the medical student, say, compressed the urethra between the speculum and the pelvic bone in a way that would cause pain to a living body. Living tissue simply feels different. It requires more subtle palpation techniques. It requires attending to what one is feeling in one's own body to understand another's body. The pelvic simulator, by nature of its design, alters the sensations in a trainee's body that are necessary for doing a comfortable exam. It alters the intra-active nature of feeling with for the medical student. These are the consequences at the level of the body of the larger debates I outlined in chapters 1 and 4, about the political stakes of an active and engaged GTA versus a passive human model or manikin. Medical students embody a different kind of "feeling with," which intra-actively produces a different kind of knowledge about the patient.

What these examples demonstrate is attention to sensation is important and that the real work of the pelvic exam requires "feeling with" as an intra-active mode of attention. Medical students must simultaneously feel the patient's body and their own bodies. Sensation travels within and between bodies, and modes of perception enact objects of knowledge in ways that disaggregate bodies as cohesive wholes. Attending to the circulation of sensation equips medical students with the ability to handle difference, contingency, and to adapt to the patient's particular body and the material arrangements of the clinic. In this way, feeling with is the directing of one's attention to sensations in particular, situation-dependent ways *in order to* make objects of knowledge out of previously indeterminate states of embodiment. However, this indeterminacy of sensation poses unique challenges that require different forms of translation and ways of enacting these boundaries between subject and object.

"Feeling with" as Translation

Part of the pedagogical work that GTAs do in session is to render sensation into something understandable to medical students. Sensation is the body registering the indeterminacy and immediacy of experience (Massumi 2002). A sensation, in this way, is a recognized affect, and perception is that process of recognition. However, to bring affect up to the level of language or awareness is to change affect entirely. Just as the body, upon registering some form of lived intensity, must transform this affect into sensation, embodied subjects must translate these sensations into something tangible that can be shared.

As I have noted repeatedly, learning clinical exam skills requires that medical students learn how to discern information about the body in ways that are unfamiliar and not present in other aspects of daily life. The pelvic exam requires learning to differentiate reproductive anatomy from other internal anatomy by touch only, which is much more difficult than it may seem from studying an anatomical textbook. The GTAs I spoke with frequently described palpating the internal organs as subtle or delicate. For their part, medical students tended to experience the process in a way that Stephanie described: "I've never felt a uterus before. . . . You're palpating on the stomach, you're trying to like feel through all the skin, all the stuff on top, trying to feel those different organs. Then you have the idea of what, where things are and how they feel and how it is to feel them." This remark speaks to the process of learning how to perceive the organs within the pelvis as objects of attention. Medical students may have felt their own or another's abdominal cavity before, but not with the clinical intention of locating and assessing reproductive anatomy. GTAs train medical students how to feel through the tissues, organs, muscles, bones, and flesh of the pelvis to locate, find, and *make an object of attention* out of the cervix, uterus, and ovaries. In this way, GTAs must find techniques for translating novel sensation into identifiable fixed points in the discursive formation of medical knowledge.

GTAs do this through touch and language. By guiding a medical student's hand more to the left to find the ovary or by encouraging a medical student to apply more pressure to insert the speculum, GTAs are training medical students how to use their bodies—their tactical senses—to perceive these organs. GTAs' bodies register sensation and act through touch to help medical students also register the sensations present in their own bodies. Touch becomes a concrete and nonverbal mechanism for translating affect. However, GTAs primarily use physical contact to correct students at the same time as they provide verbal instruction on the technique and their own sensate experience of that technique. As Jason, a medical student, explained, "You have to put your fingers in certain places and they'll say, 'Oh, you're not pressing hard enough.' 'You need to press deeper,' like, 'Oh, do you feel that' . . . [and] . . . during the exam they would sometimes guide your hand . . . 'do this' . . . 'try to get it on your own.'" As Jason indicates, while medical students are doing the exam, they're getting moment-by-moment feedback from the GTA about the sensations the GTA is experiencing in order to more fully and comprehensively perform the techniques of examination. Basil said:

> The set-up was interesting to me because she was in lithotomy position [in a reclined position with feet in the stirrups] with a mirror in hand so she could actually see exactly what was happening at all times. And she was coordinated enough to be able to guide our hands and our phrasing at the exact same time. So she . . . would give us instructions as to how our fingers and our hands should move across the pelvic area and then have us repeat whatever phrasing and instructions for the patient along the way.

In this way, GTAs use physical contact and language to translate their own sensations into instructions and guidance for the medical students. Touch and language become important tools for learning to feel with.

Through training and experience, GTAs develop skills to draw attention to medical students' sensory experiences during the pelvic exam. Jill, a GTA, was training to become an acupuncturist at the time of our interview, which is another occupation that requires close contact with another's body and close attention to one's own and others' bodily states. She provided an exceptionally interesting and detailed description of teaching medical students about palpation:

> It's not all together easy explaining or breaking down the physical behaviors of palpation and they're not inherently self-evident to people, either. . . . And I think one of my primary strategies . . . is the stuff around breaking down the physical behaviors of palpation. What does it mean to relax your hand? And being able to offer different physical sensations that equate [to] a relaxed hand. Making your hand heavy. Can you make your whole arm heavy, starting at the shoulder, all the way through your hand? Think of your hand as floating. Can you make your hand soft? . . . So breaking it down into the sensations that they can feel in their own body helps them relate to how to go about doing what I'm asking them to accomplish.

For Jill, then, the pelvic exam explicitly involves training medical students to attend to their bodily sensations in order to help them to develop the means of perceiving another person's body. She makes perception about a reciprocal link between the experience of one's own body and the experience of touch with another body (the object of study). This reciprocal link represents both attending *to* the body, in this case the body of the patient, and attending *with* the body by focusing on what the medical student feels in their own bodies.

Part of this work is linked to the nervousness and anxiety that many medical students experience going into the pelvic exam. As I discussed in chapters 2 and 4, this anxiety can be related to many things: perhaps the student has never seen genitals before or perhaps not in a nonsexual context; perhaps the student is scared of hurting the patient or seeming incompetent in front of their peers. Anxiety—whatever its source—is common. A number of GTAs told me that they often have to make medical students pause and relax before moving forward. During the bimanual exam, for example, which requires bending the wrist inward at an angle that can be uncomfortable for the clinically untrained, medical students may tense up through their arms, shoulders, and backs, so that their hunched and cramped positions prevent them from performing a proper exam. GTAs encourage medical students to think about the posture of their entire bodies, not just the position of their hand, and thereby make the pelvic exam about a mode of attention that encompasses the whole body.

GTAs use another interesting set of skills for translating affect, which is linking what medical students should feel in their bodies to the action that they should be undertaking. While I was working as a GTA, I registered a number of embodied metaphors that GTAs use to do this translational work. For example, the small, free-moving ovaries might feel against the fingers like "a ripple," "a fish swimming by," and so forth. GTAs used metaphors as well for the uterus. A nonpregnant uterus has some rebound to it, which should feel like "a tennis ball" or "a tomato." Likewise, a cervix that is "squishy like lips" indicates pregnancy; one that is firm but mobile "like a pencil eraser" is nonpregnant and healthy, but if it is "firm like bone," it could be diseased. The work these metaphors do is to translate similar feeling-states in the body into something recognizable to the student. All of these metaphors avoid anything that could be perceived as sexual. They are friendly and translate affect, as well as translate medical jargon into mundane human experiences.

I'd like to now offer a final and slightly different example of how feeling with operates in the GTA session. It emphasizes how attending to embodied experiences in the pelvic exam goes beyond direct tactile engagement with the body. As I said in chapter 3, a key part of training for GTAs is to performing the exam on a fully trained GTA with that person teaching the exam, as if the trainee GTA is a medical student. Anna said, "I feel like that's a key component because it lets you know how a student might be feeling. . . . If you're feeling nervous about doing the exam on someone else, well, then, good, remember that's how the student's feeling." GTAs who learn the exam themselves by doing it on another person are then encouraged to remember that experience when they are prepared to teach the exam. They use feeling with the medical student's nervousness and anxiety to inform their training.

Conversely, at one of the medical schools, GTAs invited medical students to assume the lithotomy position. Originally, GTAs at this specific school invited all of the men (on the assumption that they would not have had a pelvic exam) to assume the position. However, this practice became controversial, and now GTAs only ask for one volunteer. The GTA then asks the volunteer to narrate to the other students how it feels to be in the position. This practice arose at this particular medical school during the 1980s out of the ethos of feminist self-help and the spirit of reciprocal sharing. It provides an opportunity to experience in order to know how powerless the lithotomy position can make some people feel. Program coordinator Heather explained that "they need to see what we're going through as a male doctor, not just diving in there and doing what they've got to do without giving much thought to the other side." Program coordinator Martha likewise told me:

> Before we had the medical students do the exam, we had all of the males get up in the lithotomy position. And we did it very delicately because I didn't want it to be the message, "Oh, we're doing this to get back at you and to laugh at you," but to see how you feel lying down on an exam table with your feet in the footrests and having somebody stand over you. And then . . . we kept them flat on their back with the drape over their knees and . . . the examiner [sat] down at the end of the table and like rattle speculums . . . versus having the back of the table up and having . . . some eye contact . . . so you could actually see the person at the foot of the table.

The intention, as Martha explains, was about experience and empathy, not about "getting back" at medical students for what feminists might perceive as the sins of the medical profession. Martha wanted to have medical students experience both types of practice—old and new—in order to understand the experience of each. Drape sheets delimit visual perception, for example, splitting the patient's body into two regions of awareness (Young 1997). This allows the physician to ignore the patient's subjectivity during the exam. Having the medical student on the table experience both sitting up and lying down, with and without eye contact and draping, the disembodied sounds of the instruments, underscores the patient's embodied experience, turning the patient back into a full subject in the encounter. In this way, this is one mode of learning to feel with one's patient by literally putting oneself into the patient's position. However, it is also an example of translating affect into language, as the medical student on the table narrates for the other students the feelings of being in this position.

This technique is useful for both the individual medical student who assumes the position and the other medical students, who learn from the experience, as medical student Carolina explained.

> And they had one person volunteer to get on the table [to] feel sort of how you feel a little bit vulnerable sitting there. . . . I think it was a worthwhile exercise just kind of to like put yourself, even with your clothes on, sort of in that physical position, so you know how it feels, a little bit vulnerable to have your legs open and have a stranger kind of have reassure you. . . . I think it helps you be a little bit more sensitive to how the patient might be feeling. . . . Seeing my classmate . . . go up there like reminded me of the times that I've had the pelvic exam and I think it was a little bit useful to be like, oh, okay, remember what that feels like. It does feel a little bit vulnerable and let's be conscious of that as we begin learning how to do this exam.

The medical student on the table would also narrate the experience to the other students. These remarks demonstrate two things. The first is that even medical students who have had the pelvic exam may need prompting to connect their own experiences with the patient's experience when performing the pelvic exam for the first time.[13] Second, it demonstrates the use of experience as a type of evidence in collective learning processes (Murphy 2012). While medical students can certainly draw from their own embodied perceptions to understand the patient's experience, they don't necessarily have to if they are participating in a group learning process. Experience is thus both an individual asset and a stock of knowledge that is produced in collective encounters and can be selectively draw from by individuals.

However, this final way that feeling with operates in the GTA session also underscores its limitations. Feeling with as a mode of clinical perception is dependent upon the specific apparatus within which it circulates, in this case, the pelvic exam. The material objects and bodies involved are part of this and are, in fact, co-constitutive with discourse. While a person without a vagina can lie on a table and know what it feels like to be vulnerable in this way, this person does not inhabit a body that has historically and systematically been sexualized, dehumanized, and rendered pathological by medical discourse. The ways in which bodies accumulate affect outside of the exam matters for how participants will experience the encounter. But, furthermore, because the ways in which medical students are being trained to become attuned to their bodily sensations occurs within the context of the pelvic exam, medical discourses about bodies matter for how students (and patients) understand and make knowledge out of their perceptions. The power wielded through medical discourse thus limits the capacity of individuals to form empathetic attachments *because* it relies on histories of subordination of certain kinds of bodies.

Thus, as I've shown in this section, there are three primary strategies for translating or transducing affect in the GTA session: touch, language, and shared experience. Touch guides and transmits impressions by direct physical engagement between bodies; the shifting of modes of perception enables the enactment of subjects and objects out of body parts of whole bodies. Language attempts to lift affective intensities to the level of cognition by turning these intensities into something that can be shared. Shared experience collectivizes affective impressions and holds them in the present. In all of these forms, something is lost and something is gained. Feeling with becomes an embodied practice that shares perception of oneself and the material world within and around one's body and its parts.

Assembling Clinical Bodies

Scholarship on medical embodiment has long been dominated by the disciplinary perspective derived from Foucault's work on the clinical gaze (Armstrong 1983). However, this tradition has often been cast in tension with more phenomenological approaches (Young 1997). To put a great deal of sophisticated debates in deeply simplistic terms, these tensions raise questions about whether one *is* or *has* a body. More recently, however, perspectives have emerged that question the limits of representation (i.e., discourse, which is to say the inscription of language on the body) in theories based on discipline. At the same time, these theories about bodily experience question the primacy of the human subject in phenomenological accounts, asserting that there are more forms of material objects besides bodies that act on the world around them. Taken together, these new theories about the nature of the body and embodiment can be described as a tendency within new materialism (Coole and Frost 2010; Pitts-Taylor 2016). Drawing variously from work in the tradition of Gilles Deleuze and Felix Guattari, new materialist theories of *affect* ask not whether one *has* or *is* a body, but what the body *does*.

In *A Thousand Plateaus*, Deleuze and Guattari ask, "What can a body do?"

> We know nothing about a body until we know what it can do, in other words, what its affects are, how they can or cannot enter into composition with other affects, with the affects of another body, either to destroy that body or to be destroyed by it, either to exchange actions and passions with it or to join with it in composing a more powerful body. (1987:257)

Their work on assemblages and affect has thus prompted scholars to consider bodies as comprised of and interacting with components. These components include discursive formations, material objects, social forces and cultural practices, and emotions or affects. Recall from the introduction that I described affect as a verb: it *does* things. It is a capacity to affect and be affected by other material objects and bodies. Thinking of the body as an assemblage means considering how the various components of the assemblage *affect* one another, or have capacities to alter, shape, produce, or suppress the other components. Affect thus flows through and between the different components of a body-as-assemblage, binding it together and connecting its components to other assemblages.[14] As sociologist Nick Fox argues, "Affects specify or 'territorialise' . . . the limits of a body's capabilities—what it can do, feel and desire" (2016:68). In this way, flows of affect can become sedimented into the body as habits, tastes, impressions, and so forth. I want to emphasize this last point slightly more. Becoming attuned to novel sensations is one way in which bodies are made.[15] These new sensations layer into the body and become sedimented as habits. The affected body is thus the habituated body (Blackman 2013).

What I am offering here is a way of understanding the production of bodies in medicine, which attends to the inseparability of bodies from the meaning-making processes in which they come to matter and from the other kinds of bodies with which they interact. In this way, I argue that medical embodiment is not an individualized state or process, nor is it singular and self-contained; rather, medical embodiment is an assemblage. This means that not just bodies, but *knowledge about bodies*, are inseparable from the practices that produce them and the discourses in which they circulate. I am challenging our understanding of what a physician is here. The expertise that physicians produce and the authority they deploy in the clinic are *fundamentally a part of* their own embodiment and the embodiment of their patients.

This has several important consequences for how we understand medical embodiment. First and foremost, for medical trainees, developing embodied perception is a process of the body becoming territorialized by novel medical habits (i.e., the medical habitus I discuss in chapter 4).[16] This means that attention to sensation is central, not incidental. The perceptions that medical students acquire during training experiences such as the GTA session lay the groundwork for the embodiment of habits that will live in their bodies as trained physicians. Feeling hundreds of uteri will make both the action of doing the bimanual exam and the reflexive judgment of whether or not this particular uterus is the size it is expected to be or not habitual. And yet, the component of this judgment that is affective and intra-active means that habit is not a fixed, immovable thing once inculcated. It is modified ever so slightly each time it is deployed in concert with the situation or object that has provoked its use. In this way, feeling with is a habit that is constantly being remade as the physician's body moves, changes, and encounters new patients' bodies and medical tools. Thus, attention to sensation is a crucial aspect of medical work, not just part of the training process for medical students. I argue that attention to sensation and affect is fundamentally part of expertise in the clinic, as the experienced physician must constantly adjust to new bodily assemblages. Expertise, then, is the ability to improvise efficiently in the moment, to develop on-the-spot workarounds to established standards that don't quite fit, to "move with and be moved by" (Myers 2012) the local and specific. This is the essential work that the GTA program does for producing the next generation of physicians.

This leads me to the second implication of "feeling with" as an intra-active mode of clinical perception. The literature thus far on training perception in medical students has not fully accounted for the act of measurement that takes place during any physical examination, since the goal of the work is to judge the healthy and the normal from the diseased and the abnormal. Something must be measured: the size and shape of the uterus, the rebound of the belly, the location and quality of pain in the hip joint. What "feeling with" allows for in this examination of perception is an understanding of how bodies (human and nonhuman) collectively co-produce the event to be understood. Furthermore, the material objects of medicine and discourses of medical knowledge iteratively co-produce these events. Where there is no medicalized knowledge of fibroids, there is no enlarged uterus, and vice versa. Likewise, the apparatus—the particular context or type of procedure—is part of this measurement process. While these insights have been recognized in terms of the technologies of medicine,[17] the role of the physician's own body has been less recognized. I claim that through feeling with, physicians' bodies become part of the judgment and decision-making process in clinical practice. This nuances the idea that the body is disappearing in the clinic and, furthermore, emphasizes affect as a part of medical work that cannot be captured by technologies of standardization.

Finally, a third implication of feeling with has to do with translation. Because affect circulates within bodies and between bodies, both human and nonhuman, affect can be felt or experienced in clinical practice without ever being "brought up" to the level of cognition or language. Focusing on these moments of translation is important for understanding the production, capture, and destruction of affect. Patients do this work of translation in describing their symptoms, and physicians do it by situating their perceptions of any given body part gathered through palpation into the language and thus the discourse of medical knowledge. I used the example of how the medical textbook *Clinical Methods: The History, Physical, and Laboratory Methods* describes significant findings: "Ordinarily [the uterus] is firm, smooth, movable, and nontender." These are translations of perception that render a felt experience of the uterus made into an object during the pelvic exam into a medical judgment of normal or abnormal. This kind of work is routine to clinical practice. Physicians palpate and percuss abdomens, move and palpate limbs, and listen to chests, all with the goal of capturing some sensation that circulates between the patient's body and their own in the material-discursive formation of medical knowledge. In this way, technologies of affect can seek to capture these in standardized, objectified forms (as signs and symptoms under the medical gaze), but some aspects are lost or unrecognizable to such technologies. In the next chapter, I explore how medical students learn to empathize and feel with their patients under discourses of patient empowerment in medical education.

6

Not Just Bones, Organs, and Science

The New Clinical Subjects of Patient Empowerment

Early on in my research, I noticed that I was hearing a lot about patient empowerment and centering "the patient experience" in the clinical encounter from all three groups of stakeholders. This was perhaps less surprising to hear from GTAs, but I took note when I began to hear it from students and faculty. In fact, all three of the medical schools I studied are part of a national trend toward including patient-centered principles in their core competencies or by offering tracks within the general curriculum (Bensing 2000). I met one medical faculty member doing this work, Sakura, in her office in her medical school's simulation center. At the time, she was the director of clinical skills education and oversaw the "learning to doctor" curriculum for all of the pre-clerkship (i.e., first- and second-year) medical students. She shared several documents with me, including the objectives for the professionalism coursework, the rubrics used to evaluate students working with simulated patients and GTAs, and her medical school's stated values about professionalism. All of these documents emphasized taking a "patient-centered" approach. Not surprisingly, when I later interviewed medical students from this school, many of them spoke to me about the problems of "paternalistic medicine" and the benefits of "patient-centered medicine" (their words, not mine). Like almost all medical students whom I interviewed, they were enthusiastic about how the GTA session had given them the opportunity to learn from the patient experience. These students—at least in their second year of medical training—had certainly internalized the values that the school and faculty members such as Sakura espoused.

According to Sakura, this internalization process begins when students work with simulated patients—but especially GTAs.

It's hard to think of another topic in medical education where laypeople have been as successful at integrating into medical education as GTAs have. I mean I cannot think of another instance . . . we have groups of patients who have physical disabilities, who come in and talk to our students during their communication course about what is it like to live with a physical disability. . . . But that has not integrated itself into kind of the regular medical curriculum the way GTAs have. And it is just astounding how successful it's been. . . . When it starts in the individual level, you know, working with a GTA has a huge emotional impact on a student, right? Students never forget this experience. I remember the GTA I worked with almost twenty years ago. . . . And then that . . . permeates the culture and it truly is a real patient-centered educational technique. . . . I do not think you can find another example in medical education that is this well integrated. . . . Why is that? . . . I don't know, just a force of will with the GTAs and their movement and organization and . . . the willingness to work with the medical schools and adapt.

Talking to Sakura and placing the GTA session in context of the larger culture of professionalism, with its distinct norms and values, made it clear to me how this one-off experience that medical students have reflects a broader shift in the regimes of affect in medical education. Patient empowerment is a value, and today's medical students are trained to partner with their patients in a whole new range of ways.

Sakura cites GTAs' "force of will" and "willingness to work with medical schools" as one of the reasons for their long-term success in "integrating" into medical education so thoroughly. I described this in chapter 1 as a process of cooptation, and in this chapter, I pursue this theme in showing how today's technologies of patient empowerment have been shaped by the legacy of medical education research appropriating principles of feminist activism and care. I want to be very clear here: Sakura, her students, and those like her are certainly motivated by altruism and a desire to develop genuine connections with their patients. This was one of the primary things I was struck by in my conversations with them. And yet, these efforts to develop caring relationships with patients and to engage in practices of patient empowerment are situated within a structural context of corporatized healthcare. Individual physicians may care, but capitalism cares for no one. This larger structure is bound up within the strategies of affective governance in medical education that I have outlined throughout this book. Such regimes produce technologies for disciplining and shaping the conduct of those who circulate within their systems of knowledge and power.

In this chapter, I argue that patient empowerment seeks to train medical students to cultivate behaviors, attitudes, and values in patients through disciplinary work done on affect. This is linked to the technologies I discuss in chapter 2, which create specific kinds of affective ties between patients and physicians to uphold professional dominance under corporatized healthcare. Because of the pelvic exam's fraught history of rendering patients as passive objects prior to the intervention of the Women's Health Movement, this exam serves as an interesting example to tease out threads of patient empowerment and professional authority. I claim that patient empowerment is a technology comprised of discourses, knowledges, and practices that constitute patients as "partners": fully informed subjects who are responsible for and obligated to participate in the maintenance of their own health. Rather than reading patient empowerment as a challenge to top-down physician authority in the physician-patient relationship, I see it as a network of power relations deployed in the physician-patient encounter, which ultimately serve to reinforce health as both the primary goal of every individual and the exclusive domain of biomedicine. I show how medical students learn to encourage patients to become actively involved with the exam and their own healthcare and, by doing so, produce patients that are more compliant with physician authority. I then consider how these regimes exclude certain patients due to their structural positions, and I conclude with some reflections on how this could be otherwise.

The Rise of Patient Empowerment

Almost since the profession's rise to prominence became deeply embedded with science and technology at the end of the nineteenth century, physicians have recognized that the objectifying nature of the clinical gaze means that the subjectivity of the patient is obfuscated. Thus, each epoch in medical education has seen its own version of a perspective that emphasizes "humanism" in medicine. While the context and content of these concerns have changed, they continue to resurface. As I demonstrated in chapter 2, in the post–World War II period, physicians began thinking and talking about "whole-person medicine" or "comprehensive medicine" as a response to concerns about the proliferation of specialties and the increasingly fragmented model of care organized around specific diseases or systems. Comprehensive medicine was "geared mainly to the restoration or achievement of sustained optimal functioning of the patient as an organism rather than mainly to the diagnosis and treatment of a specific disturbance in such functioning, i.e., an illness" (Saslow 1948:165). These positions presage more of what we would call "primary care" today, though they lay the groundwork in some ways for later transformations with regard to emotion in clinical care. These came with the 1960s and the intervention of psychiatrists.

The "whole-person medicine" approach was championed by Michael Balint, a psychiatrist whose name is still commonly used for groups in which medical trainees collectively assess their own and the patients' emotions in relationship to treatment. Balint's work during the 1950s and 1960s was motivated by a concern that the emotions of nonpsychiatric clinic patients were especially ignored, or a "no-mans'-land" in practice. His book *The Doctor, His Patient and the Illness* (1957) argued that in the context of history-taking, among other aspects of the physician-patient relationship, the physician's job is to truly *listen* to the patient, not just glean the medical information. This parallels the feminist and other social movement critiques occurring outside of medicine at this time, as I show in chapter 1. In the 1960s, Balint (1969) organized seminars during which medical students, who had been assigned to work closely with hospitalized patients receiving treatments, reported on the patients' apparent emotional experiences, as well as their *own* emotional reaction. This was an extremely novel and controversial approach, since it made the *medical students'* feelings a central focus of analysis.

At the same time as Balint was encouraging physicians to engage with their own feelings, the patient rights movement of the 1960s was laying the groundwork for a legalistic framework that shifted how physicians would interact with patients. To fully understand how far-reaching these transformations were and how much they reshaped the physician-patient relationship, it is important to truly understand what "physician-centered" medicine looked like. Christine Laine and Frank Davidoff

(1996) delineate two dimensions of clinical practice that shifted: informing the patient of the diagnosis and involving the patient in treatment. They give the example of sharing a diagnosis of cancer. In 1961, a study found that 90 percent of physicians preferred not to tell patients that they had cancer. This is exemplary of the physician-centered regime of practice. Patients were to fully trust the expertise and authority of their physicians to the extent that they should not be told their diagnoses or involved in treatment. The patient rights movement of the 1970s shifted this culture so much that by 1979, 97 percent of physicians preferred to inform patients of a cancer diagnosis (Laine and Davidoff 1996).

The term "patient-centered medicine" first appeared in the literature in 1970 (Bensing 2000). During this time, a number of court cases helped to shift practice in the clinic. Prior to this decade, courts decided based on the "physician-centered" standard, wherein the contract between physician and patient prioritized the physician's expertise and the patient's obligation to respect it. However, in 1972, *Canterbury v. Spence* changed this by shifting the standard for informed consent from what a "reasonable physician" could be expected to tell a patient to what a "reasonable patient" should be told (Laine and Davidoff 1996). In this case, a man who had been paralyzed following surgery for back pain successfully sued for damages because he had not been told of this possible risk. Other lawsuits followed, and in 1975, the American Civil Liberties Union published a patients' rights handbook: patients needed to know the information about their diagnosis and the risks associated with their treatment options in order to make the best decisions. These rights were codified in 1991 with the Patient Self-Determination Act, which mandated informed consent from a patient-centered perspective. Patients must be told that they have the right to refuse care and that they can develop advance directives that must be followed by hospitals and clinical staff. The codification of these rights into law represents in some ways the success of patient activism in the 1960s and 1970s.

As a result, in the late 1980s and early 1990s, physicians and medical educators began talking about new ways of achieving patient empowerment. The shared decision-making framework emerged at this time, along with a host of other techniques for getting to know the "whole person" in the patient or empowering the patient in clinical medicine (Anderson et al. 1995; Barry and Edgman-Levitan 2012; Charles, Gafni,

and Whelan 1997; Elwyn et al. 2012). Physicians were encouraged to explore the illness experiences of the patient—to appreciate the meaning
the patient gave the illness and the patient's feelings about it, following
the lineage of sociological work on illness narratives (Bury 1982; Williams 1984). Physicians were also encouraged to consider the patient's
understandings and experiences in their social, familial, and cultural
contexts. Medical education scholars such as Saul Weiner and Alan
Schwartz (2015) speak of this as "contextualizing care" and link it to positive health outcomes. Such techniques hearken back to the demands
for structural awareness and intervention that feminist and racial justice
movements have made since the 1960s. In making decisions about treatment, physicians are to try to "find common ground" between their own
goals and those of the patient. With the exception of narrative medicine,[1] these techniques have largely been driven by the psy-sciences. In
particular, interviewing techniques such as "motivational interviewing," which explores peoples' ambivalence toward changing their health
behaviors (Rollnick, Miller, and Butler 2008), have been adopted and
championed by psychologists for use in the clinical encounter to better
understand and mitigate patients' emotions.

The term "patient-centered" saw exponential growth in the literature
in the 1990s. In their path-breaking book *Patient-Centered Medicine*
(1995), Moira Stewart and colleagues distinguished "patient-centered"
from "disease-centered" treatment. Generally, patient-centered medicine includes two core tenets. First, the physician must "empower the
patient and share the power in the relationship" (Stewart et al. 2014:4).
Second, patient-centered medicine requires "a balance between the
subjective and objective" (Stewart et al. 2014:4). No longer is the objectifying approach of the clinical gaze or the distanced relationship of
detached concern considered acceptable. Physicians instead must pair
understandings of objective disease-based information with subjective appreciation for the patient and the experience of illness. In fact,
Stewart and her co-authors (2014:5) later developed a diagram to help
physicians develop an "integrated understanding" of the relationship
among disease, illness experience, and health, which is "unique for
each patient." This involves "weaving back and forth" through the elements of the medical history, the physical exam, and the lab results,
which comprise the objective aspects of care, and the feelings, ideas,

functions, and expectations (forming the acronym FIFE) of the patient's subjective experience. Physicians must therefore develop "self-awareness and practical wisdom" and understand the psychoanalytic concepts of "transference and countertransference" (Stewart et al. 2014:7) as they shape the physician-patient relationship. As my participants elucidate in various ways, medical training at the undergraduate, graduate, and post-graduate levels includes a range of information on patient-empowerment techniques.[2]

However, the prevalence of patient empowerment in medical education should not be taken as evidence that the profession or, indeed, healthcare systems on the whole have reorganized around the patient. Patient empowerment has not unseated the profession's long history of striving for dominance, nor has it removed the economic and scientific forces that have reshaped healthcare. I refer broadly to these forces under the rubric of "corporatization" to understand how profit-making logics have reorganized the provision of healthcare. A driver of this reorganization is the shift toward national and multinational corporations taking over ownership of hospitals and healthcare services, which has meant increased cost-containment strategies and the consolidation of individual hospitals into multi-hospital systems (Salmon 1985). Physicians' control and responsibility for individual patients have diminished, as insurers and hospital systems increasingly manage referrals, pressure physicians to spend less time with each patient, and encourage the growth of short-term facilities such as urgent care centers or even "minute clinics" (Potter and McKinlay 2005). In addition, corporate for-profit models impose new metrics and forms of quantification, including tracking twenty-one different measures of patient satisfaction to incentivize "quality" care (Piper and Tallman 2016; Westbrook, Babakus, and Grant 2014). I discuss some of these new metrics and forms of quantification in medical education research in chapter 2.

With all of these social, political, and economic forces bearing down on the medical profession, patient empowerment is thus best understood in these contexts. As sociologist Alexandra Vinson cogently argues, "In professional terms, the use of patient empowerment discourse to shape patient participation is an exercise of physician authority, and represents a mechanism by which the medical profession resists the countervailing power of patient consumerism." (2016:1376). A key aspect of Vinson's argument is that medical trainees are now taught a variety of techniques for negotiating with patients in ways that uphold patient empowerment while also achieving the physician's goals in the encounter: these include "validating a patient's emotions, ensuring the patient understands the physician's version of the problem, securing the patient's agreement to the physician's treatment plan" (2016:1375). While these techniques originate with patient-empowerment discourse, they ultimately serve to allow physicians to achieve their goals in the encounter. More importantly, they do so by equipping physicians with the skills to uphold patient empowerment while also adapting to the new corporatized landscape of professional practice. The strategies that Vinson describes and that I outline here are all suited for building and establishing relationships in the short timeframe physicians have with their patients, working with electronic health records and other new technologies in the clinical encounter, and being suitable for assessment using various satisfaction metrics.

Thus, in all of these ways, patient empowerment is bound up in forces that drive healthcare toward profit-seeking and quantification. This story shares, in many ways, the same processes of cooptation that stripped the politics of care from early GTA programs in the 1980s. Patient empowerment techniques that originated in the feminist self-help movement have filtered into the pelvic exam in ways that seek to reinforce the professional dominance of medicine and even the drive toward the politics of life itself (Rose 2009). I argue, therefore, for an understanding of patient empowerment in terms of technologies that urge medical trainees and physicians to iteratively cultivate behaviors, attitudes, and values (which Foucauldian theory calls "forms of conduct") in patients in ways that serve to foster the biopolitical stakes of medicine. A key mechanism through which conduct is shaped is the affective capacities of bodies. Understanding patient empowerment in this way aligns with my overall argument in this book about the new regime of affective governance in medical education.

Technologies of Patient Empowerment

Medical students are taught a set of patient empowerment techniques in the GTA session that have been coopted from feminist health activism in order to achieve the physician's goals in the encounter. The "good patient" of new regimes of health involves a set of behaviors, attitudes, and values that medical students learn to cultivate in order to produce those subjects who are "good patients." Drawing on a Foucauldian perspective, theorist Nikolas Rose argues that new forms of science and technology reorder our vital capacities and lives, which he calls the politics of life itself: "our growing capacities to control, manage, engineer, reshape, and modulate the very vital capacities of human beings as living creatures" (2009:3). These modifications involved a reorganization of state powers, shifting the burden of biopower to individuals' self-surveillance and the private sector. According to Rose, the opening up of new ways of living and experiencing the world made possible by scientific and technological advances do not in fact provide freedom or liberation, but instead entail a range of new technologies of the self through which individuals are increasingly required to make themselves into the right kind of subject (Rose 1993, 1998, 2009). Within clinical medicine, this means not only that patients are given the option of participating in their own healthcare, but that they are required to participate: "Activism and responsibility have now become not only desirable but virtually obligatory" (Rose 2009:147). Likewise, historian Michelle Murphy argues:

> Rather than simply compliant and obedient, the good patient, over the course of the late twentieth century, became someone who was educated enough to ensure doctors had negotiated "informed consent," and who could be her or his own advocate, as well as someone who regulated her or his own risk and "lifestyle" for the sake of good health. (2012:118)

Thus, maintaining health by self-monitoring and self-surveillance became a moral obligation. Patients become responsible for their own health-seeking behaviors as they constantly strive to maximize their embodied capacities to be productive. This process of making patients responsible for their own health becomes tied to affect when "emotions are discursively ordered and structured as objects and effects of power within a biopolitics of governmentality" (Brown 2015:120). Good patients are thus disciplined through expert work on their affects.

Clinical practice is a key site in which this production of the good patient occurs. Physicians—as intermediaries between science and patients—exercise strategies of governance in the service of biopolitics. Cultivating empowerment is one such strategy. As sociologists David Silverman and Michael Bloor observe, patient empowerment involves "the constitution of patients as particular kinds of subjects with particular kinds of attributes by the operation of specific institutional and discursive practices" (1990:7). Furthermore, they point out, "The expansion of patient-centered medicine has sometimes been conceived within the social and clinical sciences as a reform program, but the humanization of medicine may also be read as a strategy of power" (1990:14). Thus, for example, physicians encourage patients to narrate or "confess" their illnesses and then use this information to shape the patient's thoughts and feelings to comply with the physician's wishes. Along the same lines, scholars Catherine Cook and Margaret Brunton (2015) argue that using the language and techniques of patient-centered medicine, physicians exercise productive power in the care of others. In this way, communication becomes more important in the pelvic exam than technical skills. Physicians must learn ways of using language and continually renegotiating consent during the exam in such a way as to encourage patients to keep seeking the lifesaving screening tool of the Pap smear, for example.

Embodiment is a critical location where this work of internalizing power and producing oneself as a "good" subject occurs. What affect theory allows for here is an understanding of emotion not as biological or contained inside one individual body, but as a circulating force that shapes bodies and experiences. In this way, bodily capacities are produced within structures of power. In the clinic, this means that physicians actively cultivate embodied dispositions in their patients. These dispositions align with what sociologist Janet Shim (2010) calls "cultural health capital," which accounts for all of the taken-for-granted and seemingly natural dispositions that foster health-seeking behaviors.[3] Shim writes:

Cultural health capital refers to the particular repertoire of cultural skills, verbal and nonverbal competencies, and interactional styles that can influence health care interactions at a given historical moment. At present,

> specific elements of CHC may include linguistic facility, a proactive attitude toward accumulating knowledge, the ability to understand and use biomedical information, and an instrumental approach to disease management. These kinds of cognitive, attitudinal, and behavioral resources can be deployed by patients and, depending upon providers' variable responses to them, may result in more attentive and satisfying engagements with health professionals. (2010:2)

Shim develops this concept to help us understand how inequalities in health are produced in clinical interactions. This concept is especially useful because it accounts for the values and norms embodied by the physician as well as by the patient, and allows us to grasp how physicians may intentionally or unintentionally produce desirable practices in patients:

> Providers do not simply respond to the CHC that patients mobilize, but actually contribute to their capacity to do so. In the interactive give-and-take of the clinical encounter, clinicians can signal to patients and encourage them to be the kinds of actors they would like them to be. (Shim 2010:4)

Thus, a range of capacities can be cultivated by physicians through selective engagement with patients' cultural health capital and the work that patient empowerment has been made to do in upholding the professional dominance of medicine. This work, more broadly, makes up subjects who can and will act in the "right" ways under new regimes of biopolitical control. Patients become self-responsible, and physicians are trained to cultivate forms of self-responsibility in patients.

Technologies of Patient Empowerment and Affect in the GTA Program

The use of nonphysician experts in simulation was especially important for the development of the GTA program because of both feminist concerns over the dehumanization of patients and medical educators' concerns that regular clinic patients could not give feedback. As a result, there has been a discursive framing of GTA programs as being about the patient perspective. Patient empowerment is the justification for such programs and for the techniques folded into them. In my interviews, medical students, medical faculty, and GTAs all contrasted the contemporary moment of valuing patient empowerment with a historical past that did not. What is interesting is how all of my participants valued the GTA session for its affective subject-making capacities.

Sally, the medical student who first advocated for bringing GTA programs into her medical school, said, "I think we utilize GTAs now to do assessments as well as teaching, and I think that that's really an important educational advance. . . . I think the whole notion of teaching an exam from a patient perspective was mightily important and to some extent, that is retained today." Likewise, social sciences PhD faculty member Nancy emphasized the importance of GTAs for teaching about patient empowerment:

> What I really liked about [the GTA program] is that . . . patients . . . were seen as having expertise, which of course they have. Who better to give you a feedback on how you're doing a pelvic exam on me than me? . . . I think as a woman having a pelvic exam done on me and particularly a woman who's gone through a training program, I think I would have a lot of valuable information to give to medical students.

This shift away from teaching on patients as passive objects and instead incorporating trained laypeople to autonomously teach the exam without even the presence of medical faculty was seen by my participants as a shift toward patient empowerment, which constructs patients as subjects whose perspective, knowledge, and experience are valuable to include and thereby brings patients into networks of medical expertise.

Teaching from the patient perspective is *affective* in many ways. Folding patients into medical expertise reworks flows of affect to within new regimes of medical education. Program coordinator Sergei and I had the following exchange:

> KELLY: How much of an effect do you think this has had on the medical profession and on women's experiences with getting gynecological exams?
>
> SERGEI: I think it's the best thing they've [the medical profession has] done. . . . From what I've been told . . . before they used this

technique, they would examine on unconscious patients in the surgery suite. . . . Sometimes part of that was, well, we're going to march
the students in. And they don't necessarily tell the patient that. . . .
And older faculty have said to me, that's how I learned. Older people,
you know, more senior faculty. Which I think is kind of sad because
you learn and you don't appreciate the person that you're . . . I think
it just helps you solidify the humanism piece of medicine.

For Sergei, there is an inherent difference between learning on a person
who can't speak back to the trainee (and may not even know they're
being examined) and someone who can engage with the trainee. The
latter "helps . . . solidify the humanism piece of medicine."[4] Thus,
through learning on GTAs, not only are patients being made, but medical students are as well. This experience humanizes patients—and it
humanizes physicians. It creates new pathways of affect between physicians and patients. This also has a gendered component, wherein it is
women who are being made human and doing the work of humanizing
physicians.

Medical students were enthusiastic about telling me how this exam
experience helped them to become specific kinds of physicians. For example, medical student Roger told me:

There has been a trend [to create] doctors that . . . sort of treat the patients
first and respecting the patient more. So if anything I think that this [the
GTA program] sort of helps us—the students—sort of be more sensitive,
understanding in practice, before [we] actually examine a real patient. . . .
I think it is going along the line of just having like personal respect for
and consideration for patients.

In this way, the GTA session instills values about the physician-patient
relationship in medical trainees and prepares them to work with
patients. This technology of patient empowerment works because its
target and its effect is affect—"the humanism piece," "sensitivity," and
"respect and consideration." Patient empowerment is thus a disciplinary
technology of affect.

Medical students learn in this encounter how to make themselves
into "good" physicians who respect the patient and, in this way, cultivate

forms of cultural health capital in ways that serve the workings of bio-political health regimes. The key mechanism of action here is on the affective capacities of patients. In this section, I outline four processes of subject-making through patient empowerment: (1) activating the patient, (2) appreciating the patient, (3) putting the patient at ease, and (4) making the patient self-responsible. Taken together, these four processes constitute the "patient-as-partner," or the informed and active patient favored by contemporary biopolitics. In the sections that follow, I describe each of these moves and provide examples that are not only specific to the pelvic exam, but also indicative of changes in clinical practice more generally. What GTAs teach medical students becomes a kind of gold standard or ideal type, a place at which to start for all patients. These techniques assume a patient who wants to engage with the exam, know what is happening, and see what is going on.

Activating the Patient

The first process of subject-making in patient empowerment is the move toward activating the patient. This involves a range of techniques and practices to inform and involve the patient about their health or medical care. For the pelvic exam specifically, a number of techniques have been adopted from the Women's Health Movement to help shift the patient from passive object to active subject. This shift is perhaps most strongly associated with a historical transformation in clinical practice. Medical students and faculty spoke of the move away from paternalistic medicine (and most of them in fact used that word explicitly), or a model of physician authority in which the physicians knows everything and the patient must obey unquestioningly. It is by activating the patient in the encounter that the patient's subjectivities are reworked: a patient's cultural health capital can be selectively engaged by a physician only when the patient is actively using it.

As I trace throughout this chapter, the technologies of patient empowerment that have been selectively coopted from early feminist practices of the pelvic exam in the Women's Health Movement have changed very little in the interim. For example, the GTA protocols as outlined on a 1980 "script" (included in appendix B) are very much like those that were in effect in 1999, and they still guide the GTAs who walked me through their teaching step by step. One of these protocols from 1980 concerns "patient's cooperative behavior," Which involve the following:

1. Patient agrees to have head raised, which relaxes muscles and places her in a more equal position.
2. Patient agrees to become involved in exam, i.e. feeling her own uterus, nodes, or holding sheet.
3. Patient agrees to lift gown, which gives her control of exposing her body.
4. Patient becomes aware of tense muscles and learns to relax them.
5. Patient learns to control breathing, i.e. "take a depp [sic] breath."
6. Patient learns to relax her knees out to the side, i.e. "let your knees fall out to my hands."
7. Patient supports her thighs when necessary.

All of these arrangements and behaviors indicate a patient who agrees to be and is an active participant in the exam. The patient is now sitting up and looking around, which "places her in a more equal position" (that it makes her more relaxed is helpful, too, as I will discuss). The patient is also actively involved with the tools of the exam: she lifts her gown and holds the sheet that covers her knees. She even supports her own thighs if need be. In addition, the patient is also activated in terms of her relationship to her own body: she "becomes aware" of her muscles when they are tense and "learns to relax them." She "learns to control" her breathing. She "learns to relax her knees out to the side." Finally, and perhaps mostly interestingly of all, she agrees to "feel her own uterus": she is also doing the exam along with the physician. All of these steps require a patient who is actively involved, willing *and* able to undertake these patient empowerment strategies.

The techniques that were introduced during the 1980s have made activating the patient a routine part of the exam. These include, first of all, a reorganization of the spatial relationship between physician and patient. GTAs teach medical students to put the exam table back upright and position the drape sheet so that physician and patient can maintain eye contact. A variety of communication techniques broadly called "talk before touch" are also part of the process. Medical student Ted explained how talk before touch works in practice: "You talk to the patient about what you're about to do and you do it [in a] controlled clinical way . . . like you will say, you will feel my hand on the back of your thigh before you place it." This way the patient knows what is going on in each step of the exam and what its purpose is. No longer is the patient lying back and pretending the exam isn't happening the default position. Finally, in some iterations of GTA programs that I studied, medical students provide a mirror so that the patient can sit up and view their own cervix during the speculum exam if they would like. This technique harkens directly back to the politics of feminist self-help clinics, when women viewed one another's cervices. These techniques are also present in the pelvic exam checklist put forth by Association of Professors of Gynecology and Obstetrics (see appendix B), which makes the patient an active participant in the exam.

Patients are also activated through the shared decision-making framework developed within the growth of patient empowerment. Medical student Stephanie told me:

> I think that there's a lot more focus on patient autonomy, patients making their own decisions, giving patients freedom. And there's possibly a lot more respect for patients that has happened more recently in the medical community. And there's a lot more where like you can ask a patient, "What do you want to do, here are the options, what do you want?" instead of just telling the patient what they should do.

In addition to mentioning a generalized sense of respect and autonomy given to patients, Stephanie indicates a set of techniques in the encounter itself. The physician is to ask patients what *they* want and to give information so that patients can make *their own* decisions. No longer is it acceptable for a physician to instruct the patient to do as the physician expects. The patient moves from a passive recipient of orders to a decision-making partner.

Appreciating the Patient

The second process of subject-making in patient empowerment is appreciating the patient, wherein the patient's subjectivity or interiority is constituted as something to be understood or another source of data.

Silverman and Bloor (1990) and Cook and Brunton (2015) have described the new focus in the clinical encounter on including questions about the patient's thoughts and feelings as the working of pastoral power and the incitement to confession. Likewise, Vinson demonstrates how medical education today trains students in "validating a patient's emotions" (2016:1375). However, I claim that the entire constitution of the patient as a subject who has thoughts and feelings that must be included in the clinical encounter is a new phenomenon within the framework of late modern subject-making of the kind that Nikolas Rose has variously described (1993, 1998, 2009). The inner lives of patients are increasingly being opened up to technologies of power: patients' conduct is now shaped through engagement with affect. The key emotion here is trust, and the emphasis is on relationship-building.

The development of GTA programs in the 1980s marks this distinct shift in how the patient is conceptualized, as this regime of affect shifted in medical education. This conceptualization of the patient's inner life arose from the Women's Health Movement and was selectively coopted by medical educators. In the 1980 protocol, medical students are instructed that they should "inquire if she has had difficulty with previous pelvic exams" and "elicit and respond to any patient questions." The protocol further states:

> The abdominal exam provides an opportunity to build a sense of trust and rapport with the patient which makes a quality pelvic exam possible. Attention to certain interpersonal factors is useful for this purpose, recognizing that even a healthy patient has a certain amount of anxiety which interferes with her cooperation.

It is the relationship—that "sense of trust and rapport"—that makes the pelvic exam possible. Medical students are told that even a "healthy patient" will have "anxiety" that poses challenges to conducting the exam. In this way, the patient's thoughts and feelings are important, and the trainee must appreciate how the patient experiences the exam in order to make "a quality pelvic exam possible." In all of these ways then, the patient's interiority is constructed as being crucial to access in order to do the work required of the physician.

Medical faculty, students, and GTAs described in various ways how the GTA session teaches the medical student to appreciate the patient's experience. MD medical faculty member Elizabeth told me:

> I . . . think that the approach that we take makes it very much the patient-centered experience and that we constantly kind of remind the students . . . how do we make the patient more comfortable, what strategies can you do to make the patient more at ease and I think that having that kind of mindset makes the student much more prepared to sort of approach the patient in a way that is—have empathy. . . . I think it makes them a little more open to what the patient experience really is.

According to program coordinator Sergei, Elizabeth, and others who voiced a similar opinion, GTA programs prepare medical students to understand and appreciate the patient experience in the exam, which leads to their becoming more empathetic or more able to emotionally identify with or understand what the patient is feeling. As GTA Anna explained:

> The idea of the [G]TA as being an empowered lay person in many cases who knows a whole lot about this exam and is able to teach doctors [is] sending the idea that, hey, you know, women know a lot about their body. They have a lot of knowledge that you as doctors may need to figure how to access and work as a partner with them to treat their health.

Because the GTA session uses trained laypeople, ostensibly it is designed to make medical students more aware of the patient experience since the patient is teaching them the exam. Furthermore, the patient is constituted as having knowledge that the physician should be mindful of; the patient has a subjectivity and an interiority that the physician *may need to figure how to access.* Part of the physician's job, then, is to access this interior knowledge.

The idea that a patient has an interior life that the physician must seek to understand represents a new constitution of the patient's subjectivity under technologies of patient empowerment. Patients become more than objects under the medical gaze. Medical student Michelle told me, "Combining the mechanics, the physical exam skills, with the interpersonal communication skills, I think it'll make [medical students into physicians who are] more aware of the communication side of medicine and dealing with patients not as just like bones and organs and science." Bones, organs, and science matter, but patients are more than these; patients are constituted as full subjects with thoughts, feelings, and opinions that should be engaged with. The patient's subjectivity is thus a challenge.

It is through this way of making the patient's subjectivity matter that the figure of the "patient-as-partner" is brought into being. Medical student Ellie explained:

> There's a big movement in medicine . . . about having the doctor and the patient be more of a partnership. . . . You develop a . . . partnership . . . with a patient because . . . you literally have to work with the patient in order to succeed in this particular case of performing the pelvic exam. . . . We're learning patient sensitivity and we're learning to have that sort of relationship with the patient because [in] those exams you literally have to listen to the patient and work with them in order to have success.

Appreciating the patient does not mean simply listening to the patient and empathizing with the patient. It means engaging with the patient's subjectivity such that the goal of the clinical encounter is still being met: the truth of the disease must be found (Foucault 1994). According to medical student Olivia, "It's not just about you know finding the symptoms, it's about creating a relationship with them." Success in the clinical encounter is thus tied to developing a partnership with the patient. This occurs specifically and explicitly through affect: medical students must have empathy for the patient; the patient's *feelings* about the exam are what matters. Relationship-building occurs by attending to emotion. Thus, relationship-building skills are cultivated among trainees and deployed with patients to get at their secret interiority.

Putting the Patient at Ease

Tied to this constitution of the patient's subjectivity as being crucial to locating the truth of the disease and the engagement of the patient-as-partner is the move to *put the patient at ease*. Under this regime of practice, putting the patient at ease involves a complex relationship between the humanistic values of respecting patient autonomy and the scientific goal of locating the truth of the disease. Charles, the MD faculty member who institutionalized the GTA program at his medical school and has published and spoken extensively about it, told me that he spent many hours with his initial group of GTAs trying different techniques to figure out what worked best, both to make the exam easier on the patient and to help the physician discern disease from health. In this way, the patient empowerment values of connecting with the patient, listening to the patient, and being more empathetic allows physicians greater access to the "truth" of disease. Putting the patient at ease is at one level purely physical. As I was told by several interviewees, a relaxed patient is simply easier to examine. Putting the patient at ease physically and emotionally makes the physician's job easier.

This is apparent as well in the 1980 protocol, which perhaps goes into the greatest detail about putting the patient at ease:

> A relaxed, comfortable patient is essential in order to palpate her internal structures. . . . Monitor your patient's face for cues as to her comfort. Also, it is useful to monitor the patient for muscle tension. If she seems to be resisting, it helps to slow down and give her a chance to work with you instead of against you.

This is delineated even further in the instructions on verbal behavior:

1. Acknowledge patient's anxiety (i.e., "You seem nervous about this exam, and that's understandable").
2. Inquire if she has had difficulty with previous pelvic exams.
3. Assure her that you will do your best to make the exam comfortable.
4. Provide patient with rationale for need to relax.
5. Assure patient all procedures and instructions will be shown and explained.
6. Give patient permission to stop you if exam in uncomfortable.
7. Elicit verbal commitment from patient.
8. Ask if patient is as physically comfortable as possible before proceeding with exam.

9. Use appropriate level of terminology, i.e., "not too scientific and not too condescending."
10. Avoid vocabulary with sexual connotations.
11. Avoid inappropriate humor.
12. Use supportive tone of voice.

Thus, the physician must intentionally cultivate this kind of trust and relaxation from the patient in order to do a more thorough and quality exam. The physical arrangement of the exam—putting the table back upright, allowing the patient control over her drape sheet and gown—also fits this protocol.

Its principles are still very much part of the GTA program today. GTA Sylvia explained, "I think it's really important in terms of working with the students to let them know that the patient can actually help them with the exam by letting them know if anything's hurting or pinching or pulling. . . . Because it's really helping both—really helping the practitioner, as well as the patient." I heard this over and over from GTAs and medical faculty. Learning to put the patient at ease helps the patient, but it also helps the physician. Since pain can be a sign of not only of improper technique but also of disease or pathology, a patient who is involved in the exam can assist the physician in locating disease.

While putting the patient at ease helps with the physical parts of the exam, it also helps the communication or emotional aspects of the exam. The patient-as-partner comes to trust her physician more and reveal more information about her interior life. Medical student Avery said:

> I think that it [patient-centered medicine] all comes together to help us have better communication techniques with our patients. . . . We're able to make our patients more comfortable and we're going to be able to help them more because now we are going to open up a little bit more and tell us more about what we need to more or trust us more.

Medical student Samuel likewise homed in on trust as an important resource:

> I think when the patient feels like my physician is someone I trust then they feel almost like friends, then it makes it easier for them to tell you

things, like you're going to get more meaningful information like when a patient wants to come in with some kind of symptom it might be related to some new stress at their job that you might never find out about.

For Avery, Samuel, and other medical students and faculty who spoke similarly of putting the patient at ease in this way, developing a trusting or friendly relationship makes the patient "open up" and reveal additional information about herself. In Samuel's example, being friendly with the patient might encourage the patient to provide details about a health condition related not to a physical problem, but to a subjective problem of stress or other emotion. A patient who has been put at ease is thus both easier to examine physically and more likely to share information that will make the job of the physician easier.

Thus, putting the patient at ease becomes a technology of power that produces patients-as-partners and as disciplined subjects. Medical student Olivia said:

> So I feel like introducing a program like this [GTA program] just makes better doctors . . . more sensitive to patients feelings and the patient's wants rather than kind of the hierarchical I'm the physician and you're the patient and I can do whatever I want to your body. . . . I think it just puts the patient at ease and makes them more likely to trust you, more likely to talk to you and be kind of *the ideal patients* . . . Just the ideal patient that I think would be more cooperative, they'll trust you, they'll be more likely to take recommendations for treatment, be more likely to return . . . [be] *more compliant* and . . . *easier to work with.* (Emphasis added.)

A patient whom a medical student or physician learns to put at ease becomes an *ideal* patient. These technologies of patient empowerment thus discipline patients in certain ways to serve the goals of the physician and align the patient with the workings of biopolitics in the clinical encounter. In this way, feminist challenges to the hierarchical and patriarchal authority of the medical profession become strategies for assuring patient compliance.

These dynamics are bound up in the broader political and legal climate of the practice of medicine. Cultivating an ideal patient allows the physician to get closer to the truth of the disease and produce a more compliant and docile patient, which in turn removes some of the risk of practicing in an increasingly legalistic and consumer-driven climate. In my informal discussions with GTAs, I sometimes heard them frame their encouragement of students to respect patients as "keeping them out of the courts": a trustworthy physician is less likely to be sued. As medical student Jason said:

> I think you need to be professional. . . . You have to ask about things like . . . sex and drugs and alcohol abuse . . . But at the same time to have the empathy and caring that you have to put into it. . . . People don't like doctors that don't listen to them. . . . [Doctors who don't listen] get sued . . . way more even if it's not their fault. . . . You're much less likely to get sued if you know your patient likes you, if you're available for them.

The idea that likeable physicians who listen do not get sued as often serves as a powerful lesson for medical students about the utility of putting the patient at ease. Do it because it is the right thing to do, the human thing, but do it to help yourself and protect yourself, too. And, indeed, evidence does suggest that physicians who have better communication skills and spend more time with their patients are less likely to be sued (Levinson et al. 1997). This takes the "reciprocal sharing" model of 1970s feminism and turns it into a strategy for avoiding personal and institutional harm. Such a reframing undercuts listening as a form of empathetic engagement. In this way, putting the patient at ease activates a discursive formation about trust, biopolitics, and risk that situates "bad" physicians as being in legal jeopardy.

Making the Patient Self-Responsible

The disciplining of the patient into the patient-as-partner not only makes the physician's job easier in the temporal bounds of the clinical encounter, but also extends into the future by making patients into biomedical subjects more broadly construed. Under biomedicalization, patients are responsibilized, meaning that they take the physician's job of surveillance into their own bodies.

During the GTA session, medical students learn techniques to encourage patients to continue to make regular appointments for their pelvic exams. Medical student Avery explained: "[The GTA] said that . . . this is often a good time to educate our patients. So like if you're performing a Pap smear, tell them what a Pap smear is, like explain that it's a test for cervical cancer and that it's good because cervical cancer is highly treatable when it's caught early." What Avery is referring to is a particular speech that GTAs give about training patients to keep coming back for the Pap smear. GTAs teach medical students to explain that a Pap smear is a routine screening for cervical cancer that must be performed on a regular basis in order to detect cellular changes to the cervix and prevent these from becoming cervical cancer. GTAs emphasize the idea of conveying that cervical cancer is *easily treatable* if and only if *caught early*. I've heard one or two GTAs comment informally that it is helpful to "scare" the patient a little into coming back. I find the use of fear as an interesting tactic, since it engages other forms of affect that motivate patients to see physicians. This technique attempts to construct the physician as a trustworthy ally against risks of death and disease: cancer is scary, but your physician can help you avoid it *if* you comply with regular screenings. In some ways, this evokes older, more paternalistic models of the physician-patient relationship, in which a patient is a wayward child in need of guidance from an authority figure. Moreover, this technique of explaining the importance of Pap smears frames patients who do not get them as uneducated about their importance, rather than unable due to lack of access to healthcare.

Though it has become controversial and GTAs note that not every hospital or clinic will encourage this, GTAs also train medical students how to teach patients about the breast self-exam. Guidelines changed while I was conducting this research, after several studies demonstrated that breast self-exams were not beneficial for detecting breast cancer and in fact increased false positives and "unnecessary" medical visits (Oeffinger et al. 2015). Instead of teaching medical students to always instruct patients on a full breast self-exam, GTAs now teach medical students about "breast awareness," which means being aware of any changes between their breasts or changes over time, and to emphasize the importance of explaining risk and clinical screening guidelines to patients.

This shifts the burden of responsibility for patients from actively monitoring their bodies to being aware of their risk for breast cancer and acting accordingly to get mammograms.

Such educational movements link technologies of patient empowerment with active, involved patients who take charge of their healthcare. GTA Sylvia said:

> I think it is empowering for the patient to come in the room and to be working with an examiner who acknowledges them as having some awareness of their own body. And actually to be empowering for that woman in that experience. . . . I often talked to my students about using the exam as an opportunity to educate the patient about their own self-care as well. . . . You can use that time more constructively to talk with your patient about how she can take care of herself and her own needs. . . . And it's a way of eliciting more information as well as helping your patient to take more responsibility for her own health.

In fact, the whole purpose of many of the techniques GTAs teach is to empower patients with knowledge about their own bodies. These techniques harken back to the Women's Health Movement. Offering a mirror, for example, allows patients to learn what their genitals look like so that they can monitor their genitals for changes. Allowing patients to feel their own uteri informs patients about their bodies: is their uterus tipped forward or backward (anteverted or retroverted)? Such types of self-empowerment have thus become coopted by efforts in biomedicine to make patients responsible for their own health and risk (Murphy 2012).

In this way, what GTAs teach medical students how to shape patients' subjectivities. GTAs encourage medical students to contribute to a biomedical disciplining of patients as active and self-responsible. Ideal patients don't simply come into the clinic on a regular basis and submit to biomedical authority; they are informed and active in their own healthcare. By teaching medical students how to encourage self-monitoring practices like the breast self-exam, monitoring the genitals for changes, and knowing what a Pap smear is and does, GTAs contribute to making patients self-responsible. Through biomedical education in the clinical exam, a patient "can take care of herself" and "take more responsibility for her own health." But, unlike the self-help clinics where these techniques were developed, such efforts to make patients self-responsible only further enfolds them into biomedical power. Patients monitor their bodies not to treat themselves, but to know when to visit their physicians.

Cultivating Health Capital through Technologies of Patient Empowerment

Thus, through all four of these processes of iterative subject-making in the GTA session, medical students are taught to cultivate the forms of cultural health capital most valued under current biopolitical regimes of health. In doing so, medical students' own selves are crafted so that they can most effectively engage with patients who have these valued forms of "good patient" subjectivity. This process occurs through the modification and manipulation of affective capacities of medical students and patients. To be an empathetic, patient-centered physician is to adopt a kind of affective disposition that is trained into the body. Likewise, an active, self-responsible patient is created through disciplinary work on affective capacities for the purposes of cultivating trust, relaxation, engagement, attention.

The ways in which medical students are taught to cultivate patient empowerment here are tied to larger trends in medical education research. Thus, on the United States Medical Licensing Exam Step 2, clinical skills (CS), which all physicians must pass to be licensed to practice, trainees are specifically scored on "the patient-centered communication skills of fostering the relationship, gathering information, providing information, helping the patient make decisions about next steps and supporting emotions" (Federation of State Medical Boards of the United States, 2018:11). While in the pelvic exam, specific techniques of patient empowerment have been coopted from the Women's Health Movement, these broad technologies demonstrate how medical education research has reworked the networks of power within the clinical encounter. Medical students and patients must be made into good subjects of biopolitical control via work on affect.

However, these technologies leave some patients out. Take as a first issue of consideration the process of activating the patient in patient-centered medicine. Here, the patient is informed and involved in decision-making every step of the way. As Shim's cultural health capital framework points out, participation in decision-making requires patients who have the kind of cultural capital that enables them to understand and apply medical knowledge and information. Likewise, the technique of appreciating the patient posits a patient that can be befriended and worked with to uncover interior truths, which will help the physician in diagnosis and treatment. Where the goal of putting patients at ease and listening to them is to create a trusting relationship, certain patients cannot be brought into the fold—namely, patients who have very good *structural* reasons for distrusting the medical profession, reasons that cannot be damped down by any amount of "talk before touch." And finally, making the patient self-responsible requires a patient who can access and exercise the technologies that produce responsibility as defined by biomedicine, such as the ability to get regular exams. In all these ways, physicians under patient empowerment draw from, foster, and respond to a form of cultural health capital that favors a particular kind of patient.

Resisting Normalizing Technologies of Patient Empowerment

While some in medical education have made the case that true patient-centered communication can reduce bias in the clinical encounter (Beach et al. 2007), others have noted that physicians are more verbally dominant, are less likely to engage in patient-centered communication, and generally tend to be less warm and friendly (display "positive affect") with Black patients (Johnson et al. 2004). It has also been observed that patients who engage in more active and self-advocating communication receive more facilitative communication from physicians (Gordon et al. 2006). Insofar as the pelvic exam is concerned, this means white, middle-class, cisgender patients in the contemporary United States. In the sociological literature on health promotion, it has also been noted that healthcare providers foster values of self-responsibility and empowerment in the patients they view as worthwhile and marginalize the patients who do not possess the appropriate cultural health capital.[5] The assumption that Black patients cannot fully embrace health promotion techniques surely motivates white physicians to dominate the conversation, even as the legacy of medical racism surely makes it even more difficult for Black patients to embrace communication techniques that rely on trust and warmth with white physicians.

How might we make sense of these regimes of exclusion, wherein marginalized patients are not captured by technologies of empowerment? How do these technologies—which are embedded in medical education with the intention of equalizing power in the clinical encounter—actually instead reproduce unequal relationships? Critics of biomedicine working in a neo-Foucauldian tradition have noted that biopower is unevenly applied. Those who are "made to live" and those that are "let die" are different populations. The kinds of technologies of the self that make one into the ideal biomedical subject are unevenly accessible because of structural positioning (Decoteau 2013; McCabe 2016; Sweet 2018). To examine what technologies are embedded in patient empowerment to produce the "ideal patient" demands an articulation of their values and norms, as well as to ask what forms of exclusion place becoming self-responsible out of reach for certain subjects (Sointu 2017).

I want to think carefully about how technologies of affect like patient empowerment—and all the norms and values embedded in them—produce some subjects as "ideal" and render others as targets for either exclusion or disciplinary regimes of control. Affect has everything to do with this process, as both the target of technologies and as a social marker that always already inscribes bodies with value (Clough and Halley 2007). The bodies of some patients under new regimes of affect in medical education are marked as valuable: their affects are catered to, managed, and extracted via metrics such as patient satisfaction scores in order to produce value for corporate hospital systems. Other bodies are excluded or subject to more direct regimes of governmentality that ignore their feelings and subjectivities.

How might we imagine resistance to these normalizing forces? I offer three possibilities that might produce more equitable physician-patient relationships. I am inspired in this work by the original aims of the Pelvic Teaching Program. Their revised protocol made several demands of medical education to rework its economic, political, and cultural structures of domination. How might we rethink simulated patient programs such as the GTA session that purport to be about "the patient experience" in ways that uphold and affirm normalizing forces of biopolitics and affective governance in medical education and thereby marginalize some patients?

Medical students themselves are engaging in resistance, by organizing protest against the increasingly expensive and complex forms of simulation used to evaluate their performance. At the time of this writing, over 18,000 medical students had signed onto a petition called "End Step 2 CS," which leverages the extraordinarily high cost of this test ($1,275 per attempt) and its overwhelming pass rate (95 percent) to demand an end to this portion of the USMLE (Anon. n.d.; Okwerekwu 2016). It is unclear yet what effect this kind of organized protest will have, but it should be taken as evidence that medical students themselves are pushing back against the expensive, time-consuming, and metric-driven ways in which their affective capacities are being captured by the machinery of medical education research. It is very interesting to note that this kind of massive resistance is not being demonstrated toward purely experiential forms of learning with simulated patients. As I outlined in chapter 4, when medical schools have attempted to cut GTA programs, students have complained. This kind of standards-dictated simulation of communication skills is somewhat unique to the United States context. This is in part because the United States is one of only a handful of countries (along with Canada and most southeast Asian countries) that requires a national licensing exam in the form of the USMLE (meaning, with a standardized clinical skills component), though calls for their implementation in Europe and especially the United Kingdom are increasing (Rizwan et al. n.d.; Swanson and Roberts 2016).[6] At the same time, debates about the effectiveness of such national licensing exams are mounting, with some claiming that there is limited evidence to support their validity (Archer et al. 2016; Price et al. 2018). In many European countries, simulated patients are used more for "formative" education, meaning exploration, skills-building, and experiential learning (Cantillon et al. 2010). Medical schools in the United States should thus endeavor to develop more patient-driven simulation that is not linked to testing and licensing. Today's medical students face so many unique challenges in the clinical context, and the proliferation of standards-driven simulation will likely only continue to turn positive projects such as patient empowerment into normalizing "teach-to-the-test"–style discipline.

Second, there is an ever-present challenge in expanding simulated patient workshops such as the GTA program to incorporate forms of patient subjectivity previously excluded by biopolitical regimes. As I outlined in chapter 1, even as these types of workshops can produce changes at the margins of medical practice, there is always the danger that medical education will coopt the skills and techniques taught in them. And yet, it cannot be ignored that the GTA program *has* reworked the provision of care. Given this, I am interested in how other health-care workers are adapting simulated patient programs to meet the needs of previously excluded and marginalized patients. For example, there are queer-focused GTA organizations that provide pelvic and genito-urinary exam instruction to healthcare providers in a way that empha-sizes gender-affirming skills (MacFife 2019). These and other programs that expand the kinds of patient bodies that medical students learn from are important to push back against normalizing forces of biomedicine. Seeing historically marginalized patients as *experts* could offer tremen-dous benefits. Likewise, I am curious how we might adapt simulation technologies to meet the needs of marginalized *physicians*. What would a simulation workshop that helps trainees practice dealing with sexist or racist microaggressions in the clinic look like? How might experiential training programs that use simulation be leveraged to help physicians learn how to assist marginalized patients in navigating *structural* sys-tems that disempower them? Could we see, for example, a situation in which a GTA session is used to help physicians learn how to screen and manage housing instability among transgender men of color? Break-ing simulation out of its standards-driven track could serve to open up spaces where other forms of empowerment are possible.

Finally, GTA programs aren't the only ways in which medical stu-dents interact with patients who are teaching them about the patient ex-perience. Patient navigators and other educational models help medical students to experience what it is like to live, for example, with a chronic illness as they follow a patient from appointment to appointment over the course of weeks or months (Henry-Tillman et al. 2002). How can we think about the teaching that these patients do and that GTAs do as forms of caring commitments instead of as work that develops medi-cal students' abilities to "handle" patient challenges? Instead of test-ing and measuring students' empathy in a myriad of new and complex ways, could we instead value the qualitative experience of being with patients—moving with and being moved by them? GTA programs have succeeded in part because of GTAs' force of will, yes, but maybe also because they provide caring commitments to and with medical students in an otherwise objectified curriculum. In talking to GTAs, I am always struck by their desire to improve healthcare, even to the point of putting the intimate interiors of their bodies on the line to do so. And when I speak to medical students and faculty, I recognize the motivation to care for and about patients, even as these desires are caught up in the science-oriented work of medical education research to produce objective measures of trainee performance and the for-profit pursuit of corporate healthcare.

These are pressing questions, since as I write this, there is a proliferation of concern around burnout among physicians. Technologies of affect are multiplying in order to manage this seeming crisis and prevent its serious consequences, up to and including physician suicide. And yet a small but growing number of critics within and outside of medical education are calling attention to the *structures* that produce inequality. Corporatized healthcare does not care about people, only profit. Developing technologies that will only aid in extracting more affective value out of physicians will do little to solve this problem. Instead, we need to build structures that support caring commitments within and against regimes of affective governance in medical education. Perhaps burnout is a form of resistance against a system designed to extract the maximum amount of value from one's caring labors, and perhaps to keep on caring in spite of this is as well.

Conclusion

Is the Vagina Different from the Mouth? Affect and the Making of Physicians

Every few years, a scandal reemerges in medical education: medical students perform pelvic exams on anesthetized patients without their approval. A 2003 study launched a controversy when it demonstrated that clerkship students were commonly—up to 90 percent of them—asked to perform such exams (Ubel, Jepson, and Silver-Isenstadt 2003). A report by a group of medical students in 2010 provoked fury in the media. Most recently—at least, as I write this—the popular National Public Radio program *This American Life* aired an episode about this common practice.[1] The episode "But That's What Happened," aired originally on November 9, 2018, interviews bioethicist Phoebe Friesen, who published an article in *Bioethics* on the importance of informed consent before doing pelvic exams on anesthetized patients. In her interview with *This American Life*, Friesen reports that she wrote the article after she began teaching bioethics to medical students and became aware of just how many of them were doing these types of exams: "As long as they were participating in gynecological surgeries, it was really the norm." Many of these students were emotionally conflicted about the practice: "A lot of them felt kind of confused or maybe ashamed" (National Public Radio 2018).

Given that GTA programs have been the norm in medical education since the mid-1980s, how does something like this still happen? While all patients at teaching hospitals in the United States sign a consent document prior to surgery allowing medical students to participate in their care, many are not told that they might be examined by said medical students or do not meet them before going under anesthesia. When this occurs, it is usually in the context of gynecological surgery, when a patient has some sort of pathology that a medical student would otherwise not have the opportunity to feel during a regular exam in the clinic.

This practice is receiving renewed attention—and outrage. In Chicago, where I studied teaching and learning the pelvic exam, two law professors wrote a commentary in the *Chicago Tribune* arguing: "Stop treating unconscious female patients like cadavers" (Wilson and Kreis 2018). Invoking #MeToo, the powerful movement against sexual assault, they demanded that fully informed consent always be obtained before medical students examine unconscious patients: "It is time to treat women like adults. It is time to #JustAsk." Their critiques echoed those raised by feminist activists in the 1960s and 1970s: patients are not passive objects for students' use, and a pelvic exam without consent is rape (Kapsalis 1997). Reactions to the article circulating online evoked two sorts of responses. The first included outrage and demands that such practices be banned. The second involved puzzlement and indifference since this practice is business as usual for medical professionals. These tensions reflect centuries-old debates within the profession about increasing medical knowledge for the public good versus the welfare or rights of individual patients.

One of the reasons given to justify this common practice is that a vaginal exam is no different than other kinds of exams. Friesen calls this the "Is the vagina different from the mouth?" objection. As this argument goes, medical professionals are trained to view the reproductive organs as no different from any other part of the body and to render every aspect of the body into an object that evokes no emotional reaction from them. And, indeed, medical students routinely participate in all kinds of surgeries, in which they examine the insides of bodies to gain more knowledge. While this may be all well and good for the physician, Friesen claims that the bioethics of the situation demands that the physician understand the patient's perspective.

> The important point here is that the relevant perspective with regard to determining what is trivial is that of the rights-holder, not that of the medical student or clinician. . . . It is easy to see that we ought to defer to the patient's own understanding of what is significant, not that of the physician, in order to prevent violations of trust and to promote trustworthy acting. (2018:306)

Likewise, in her interview with *This American Life*, physician Sara Wainberg—who wrote the above-mentioned study in 2010 as a medical student—argues:

> So who cares? This is just another exam. This is just another thing that medical students do in the hospital. Why is it different than looking in someone's mouth, or looking at their hip? How is this different? . . . The thing that really makes it different is not what we, as doctors, think about it. The thing that makes it different is what the patients think about it. And if you ask women, they think it's different. . . . For me, I would want to know if somebody was going to be examining my vagina while I was asleep . . . I've been there. I've been that crying woman waiting to go into surgery. So I understand what it feels like. (National Public Radio 2018)

Here, we see affect moving between the bodies of physicians and patients, attaching variously to body parts (is the vagina different from the mouth?) or residing within bodies (as discomfort or ease with pelvic exams on unconscious patients). As these affects circulate, they accumulate value, and their value is felt or deployed in different ways (as arguments for or against this practice). Thus, affects can be deployed to uphold the status quo or used in resistance. In this case, both medical students and patients harness anger, sorrow, disgust, and fear to critique this common practice. For medical students, their discomfort can sometimes be so great that it prompts them to question their superiors or launch studies at the risk of their careers to expose the practice. For bioethicists, educators, and patient advocates, what the experience *feels like* for patients underpins the whole rights-bearing apparatus that demands informed consent. Affect therefore circulates, shapes embodied encounters, and has instrumental use.

Thus, affect can be mobilized for change (Gould 2009). In affective economies, emotions are leveraged to make political claims (Ahmed 2004; Buchbinder and Timmermans 2014)—emotions *do* things. Organized resistance to these practices by medical professionals has helped usher in laws against unapproved pelvic exams during surgery in at least six states. Professional associations such as the American Medical Association, the Association of American Medical Colleges, and the Association of Professors of Gynecology and Obstetrics have issued resolutions against the practice (Adashi 2019). Indeed, as these debates intensify, GTA programs are receiving more attention and are being posited by some in the medical profession as a valuable and necessary solution (Tsai 2019), bringing core tenets of feminist health activism from the 1960s and 1970s into the current historical movement. Then, as now, affect is an unruly and disruptive force, and collective action can create change.

I am interested in what these debates about the role of consent in teaching and learning the pelvic exam can teach us about affective governance in medical education and the making of physicians. The presence of the GTA program in most medical schools in the United States has meant an enthusiastic embracing of the "patient experience." And yet, as the above debate demonstrates, there is still a prioritization of the learning experience of the trainee at the expense of the patient. That critics demand that medical schools "stop treating patients like cadavers" seemingly affirms the idea that for all of the advancements made in medical education toward fostering empathy and supporting patients' autonomy, the physician-patient relationship is still fundamentally a one-sided practice of objectification.

How are today's medical students to make sense of the fact that they are painstakingly taught and tested on their ability to use the correct language and forms of touch—all the things one medical student I interviewed criticized as the "finesse" of the exam—and then also left alone to perform a pelvic exam on an unconscious and likely not-consenting patient? What messages do medical students take away about interacting with patients from these experiences? What do they learn about when and how to utilize empathy? Is empathy more than a strategy for obtaining patient compliance? Conversations with passionate medical educators and physicians reveal that empathy is highly valuable to their work, not just for rote purposes, but for keeping them human. And yet, what else is going on here, other than that emotions and affects are valued differently in different clinical spaces and deployed for divergent purposes? What can thinking about affective governance in medical education help us understand about what it means to make good physicians?

From the rise of empathy metrics to the routinization of mindfulness practices, affect is being produced, harnessed, and managed in new and increasingly complex ways. The feelings of patients and physicians are being used to support, defend, or attack the professional dominance of medicine in novel and contradictory ways. The value of affect is produced thus by forms of expertise. Certainly, there is nothing new about the fact that medical students are trained to care about patients in specific and professionally delimited ways. There is nothing new here in the tension between extending care and dictating treatment. There is nothing new about the quest to find the human or humanism in medicine. But what is new is the ways in which these dynamics play out. The intentionality and intensiveness of technologies of affect are new, even as their purpose—the articulation of professional dominance—is not. I see these new technologies related to older modes of emotional socialization in the way I see the relationship between medicalization biomedicalization. These technologies of affect are multi-sited, multi-directional; they work from the inside out. They involve a transformation from the sovereignty of the medical profession to new visions of inter-professionalism in practice and training. They involve intensive crafting of the self, which relies on incorporations of ever-more sophisticated scientific knowledges from psychology and education. They involve all of these elements working in concert in the name of producing health.

And yet, what is not new is the quest for professional dominance and the moral value of health itself. Moreover, what is not new is the capitalist exploitation of the worker. In the strictest sense, what I argue about affective governance in medical education is that it is about producing better, more efficient workers, and more active, compliant consumers. In short, it is no longer possible to set aside the important role that emotion and bodily capacities to "move and be moved by" play in the governance of conduct via expert knowledge.

In describing the work of specially trained simulated patients known as gynecological teaching associates, who teach medical students the pelvic exam, I have considered new modes of emotional socialization in medical education. I have shown how many of the valued communication skills and their standardization, as in the checklist, come from medical education research, itself a distinct body of expertise focused on producing the next generation of physicians. I have also shown how the rise of medical education research has changed medical training and, specifically, teaching and learning the pelvic exam. The work GTAs do is a specialized form of intimate labor, in which they use their own bodies to produce affective ties between medical students and future patients and allow medical students to practice the emotional and affective dispositions of professionalism, which I have called the medical habitus. Simulation in this way also allows medical students to develop the sensorial capacities to physically examine patients. Teaching and learning the pelvic exam is guided by discourses about patient empowerment, which teaches medical students how to subtly guide patients' behavior in order to maximize their health-seeking capacities.

In all of this discussion, I have advanced a concept of technologies of affect to understand knowledges, practices, techniques, and discourses that seek to produce community, connectivity, and other bodily capacities to engage with and be affected by others. I have explicitly named and implicitly discussed several different technologies, which I see as proliferating in medical education today. I have discussed simulation, the communication checklist, and patient empowerment as specific examples. Throughout the book, though, simulation is primarily the technology of affect that I am concerned with, and I see it as a major vehicle for the modification and transmission of affective states and intensities in medical education and health professions training more broadly. Simulation is developed out of scientific bodies of knowledge about technique and interpersonal skills, and it transmits the norms, values, and attitudes of the profession as a whole through explicit and implicit lessons about best practices. It involves a production of affect by a skilled worker and the modification of the affective capacities of a trainee. Simulation is now a major way in which trainees in the health professions learn how to do their jobs.

It has not, however, entirely replaced practicing on real patients, nor in some cases should it. Clinical rotations are still a major and important training ground for medical students to learn about patient care and embody the values of the profession. In the case of the pelvic exam, physicians are still making arguments that medical students need to practice their skills on patients who are under anesthesia in order to fully appreciate gynecological pathology (Wolfberg 2007). Most medical schools in the United States today use a hybrid method, involving manikins, GTAs, and real patients, with 72 percent of schools using GTAs (Dugoff et al. 2016). Internationally, GTAs are used in Canada, Australia, and parts of Scandinavia, and they have been introduced in the United Kingdom and Turkey (Janjua et al. 2017; Sarmasoglu et al. 2016; Smith et al. 2015). Thus, while practicing on real patients is still a major component of medical training, simulation is extremely common and often the first step toward working with real patients. In this way, even if in the big picture it is only a small part of training, it is a foundational one, and it is part of a larger assemblage of practices that harness and manage affective capacities.

There are other technologies of affect in medical education today, and many others in the health professions more broadly. As healthcare is increasingly subjected to forces of privatization and neoliberalism in the United States and, indeed, abroad, as scholars in the United Kingdom and elsewhere have noted (Maynard and Williams 2018), the ways in which workers are produced to will continue to change. As I see it, given the intensifying discussions and proliferation of discourse about burnout among the professions, even at the same time as low-status care workers have taken the spotlight in some circles, these technologies of affect will only multiply.

Why Affect, Why Now: Affect and Control in Late Modern Capitalism

I have distinguished affect from emotion throughout this book. I have also used affect to describe several different phenomena, and I would like to clarify the "multiple lives of affect" (Holzberg 2018) at work in this book. My primary notion of affect comes from the Deleuzian tradition to understand affect as a pre-social, pre-linguistic impulse lived at the level of the body, as a sort of intensity or "becoming" that enables connections and closures. Affect is the capacity to sense, to relate, to form connections, to moved or be moved by objects (Murphy 2012; Myers 2012). Affect doesn't reside in individual bodies, but rather gains its effects through circulation. In this way, my discussion of sensation and perception is perhaps the clearest case of this form of affect. However, my broader framing of the tension in medical education between scientific ways of knowing and affect also relies on understanding affect as a bodily capacity. In my discussion of the checklist, for example, I have indicated how bodily intensities that enable relationality in the clinical encounter (such as empathy and compassion) are beyond what can be captured by language and thus evade efforts to produce standardized measurements and instruments. In this way, affect always already partially escapes attempts to contain or harness it within technologies of power. This means that resistance to technologies of power can be found both in the agency of individuals and in the unexpected connections formed through affective intensities.

A second way in which I have used affect comes from the literatures on affective labor, which think about new forms of work that involve immaterial labor, or the production of affects in the service of the constant creation of capital for capital's sake. These literatures build upon understandings of emotional labor, which consider workers' management of their own emotions to produce an experience or a sense of connection *between* worker and client. In this way, my analysis of the work of relating to patients and building trust in the clinical encounter relies on this reading of affective labor. My discussion of the use of simulated patients as a new mode of education for the health professions also involves this notion of affective labor. I wish to stress this point even more: given the rapid changes to the medical profession caused by patient consumerism, affective labor is an incredibly useful concept for understanding the new challenges faced by physicians and medical trainees. In addition, the increasing emphasis on interprofessional collaboration, which invokes and dismantles old hierarchies in the professions, can be understood as well through this lens. Here, I think of resistance in the acts of healthcare workers themselves, in their refusals of subordination, and in their efforts to infuse into their work forms of care that exist beyond the mandates of clinical empathy.

Finally, I have considered affective economies, in which affects gain their potency *through* circulation. Affective economies shape how affects are valued in a given social situation, and they "surface" the bodies of participants by attaching emotions to those bodies. My discussion of the emotional attachments to reproductive anatomy—i.e., the "sacred vagina"—invokes this form of affect as circulatory force. Affective economies in clinical medicine set the conditions for what might be felt by physicians and patients, and attach monetary and cultural forms of capital to the expression or suppression of emotional states of being. My discussion of how the feminist health movement leveraged emotion to force medicine to reshape teaching and learning the pelvic exam is an example of how affective economies can be grounds for resistance.

Drawing thus from these ways of thinking about affect, and especially the last form, I now highlight a concept that links all of these ways of understanding affect: affect as *biovalue*. A growing literature on the new bioeconomy considers "the multifarious ways that the biotechnical processes of 'life itself' are involved in networks of commercial transaction and capital accumulation" (Cooper and Waldby 2014:5). In these works, biovalue "refers to the yield of vitality produced by the biotechnical reformulation of living processes" (Waldby 2002: 310). Biovalue is often appropriated through practices such as banking of blood, sperm, umbilical cord blood, and embryonic stem cells (Annandale 2014). However, I would argue that affect is a key component in the constitution of life itself, as it involves the capacities of bodies to form attachments and impressions (Schuller 2017). Thus, thinking about affect as biovalue can account for the capital-generating strategies in clinical medicine and the health professions more generally that extract profit from the impressionability, ability to form connections, or emotional labor of health professions workers.

Writing on Foucault's unfinished work on biopower, Ben Anderson argues that biopower has two distinguishing characteristics. First, "it involves a referent object—either living beings or life itself—that requires knowledge of the processes of circulation, exchange and transformation that make up life" (2012:30). Second, "it is based around forms of intervention that aim to optimise some form of valued life against some form of threat: a productive relation of 'making life live'" (Anderson 2012:30). In Foucault's work, biopower is organized around institutional sites, through "enclosed institutions of civil society" (Clough 2003:360). And yet, the shift from disciplinary societies toward societies of control has meant a breakdown in these institutions, which has also entailed a shift in the "referent object" of biopower and the "productive relation" of interventions.

The target of control . . . aims at a never-ending modulation of moods, capacities, affects, potentialities, assembled in genetic codes, identification numbers, ratings profiles and preference listings; that is to say, bodies of data and information (including the human body as information and data). Control works at the molecular level of bodies—and not necessarily, or only, human bodies. (Clough 2003:360)

In this way, we have seen a major shift since the 1970s and 1980s in the target of biopower and the forms of life that it governs: "in the 'real subsumption of life' desires, subjectivities and needs are constantly mutating alongside capital" (Anderson 2012:33). Thus, we are seeing an emergence of a new "bioeconomy" aimed at the endless circulation of new forms of "life itself" via the production of affective capacities. Or, to put this more clearly, as I have stated elsewhere in this book, the mode of capitalist production is no longer aimed at the thing (good or service) produced by the worker's labor-power, but at the commodification and exploitation of the productive capacities of bodies. The worker is no longer in the factory making widgets for the widget store to sell. The worker is instead making people desire widgets; the worker's very body down to the molecular level is being turned into the widget itself. A similar process is occurring in the type of work performed by physicians and other healthcare professionals (Brown 2015; Ducey 2010).

We are familiar in medical sociology with understanding the emergence of these new forms of life through conceptualizations of biomedicalization. We understand pharmaceuticals as engendering new ways of thinking about ourselves and our having bodies (Bell and Figert 2012; Mamo and Fosket 2009). We have traced the global economy of clinical labor, including tissue donors or those who sell their organs, commercial surrogates and those who sell their reproductive materials, or those who participate in clinical trials (Cooper and Waldby 2014). We have written about the reproduction of biological racism through research on genetics (Nelson 2016; Wailoo, Nelson, and Lee 2012). The impact of these new forms of life cannot be understated. I want to add to thinking about biomedicalization and the governance of life itself by conceptualizing these processes through the literatures I have mentioned above on affect and control. The *potentiality* of life is increasingly being harnessed by capital, and the capacities of bodies to affect and be affected are becoming both the target of biopower *and* the mode of intervention.

I argue in this book that we cannot fully understand the contemporary state of the medical profession—in particular, training for it—without understanding how affect is a target of and mode of intervention in societies of control. Indeed, I see technologies of affect—as I have described them here and in as-yet unnamed new ways—as being the mechanism through which the medical profession now operates to guide the conduct of the public. Affective capacities of both medical professionals *and* patients are becoming the target of forms of biopower, guiding, encouraging, and creating forms of relationality and futurity. Affective capacities are likewise the mode of intervention: trust, hope, and empathy are the new mechanisms through which physicians secure patient compliance and through which patients participate in medical decision-making.

Literature on affect and control also points to "bodies of data and information" (Clough 2003) as novel targets and interventions of biopower. We can see this in the medical profession in the proliferation of metrics such as patient satisfaction scores, empathy scales, hope scales, burnout inventories. We also see it in increasingly targeted methods for tracking productivity via measuring appointment length, number of patients seen, efficiency of hand-overs, adoption of electronic health records. Bodies of data and information in the clinic are being produced alongside physicians' bodies, and patients' bodies are sources of capital. Big data is increasingly being hailed as a cutting-edge technology for clinicians to work smarter and more effectively. These technologies of affect are being produced by experts, both within and outside of medical education.

In all of these ways, then, conduct is being shaped by new bodies of expertise in order to govern "at arms' length." Modulation and modification of affect via control is making physicians more productive, even as it is changing the nature of medical work to be oriented toward the endless deployment of productivity as an end for capital in and of itself. This binds physicians and patients together, and binds them to other health professionals, bodies of data and information, and non-human bodies via new tools and technologies, through clinical work.[2] New forms of governance thus operate on and through affect and emotion, even as affect and emotion are targets of expert governance. In this way, I argue for studies of expertise that consider the affective economies in which expertise circulates, and from which expertise gains its salience.

What about Gender and Sexuality? What about Inequality?

While expertise operates through modification of affects, all experts cannot embody expertise uniformly. Because affect "surfaces" bodies, and because affect is being harnessed as target and vehicle for biopolitics, the ability to embody and use expertise is unevenly distributed across populations. We see this unevenness in the literature on communication skills by gender and race or ethnicity of trainee: in standardized tests, white women are rated mostly highly, while Black men are rated the most poorly (Berg et al. 2015). This aligns with both the historical and contemporary racism of the medical profession *and* arguments about its feminization. I suggest that affective governance produces valuations of who or what kinds of bodies can deploy expert authority. Take, for example, women in medicine. Women do better in standardized tests of communication skills and are rated more highly in tests of empathy. And yet women remain underrepresented in the higher prestige fields, where patient contact is minimal and empathy is beside the point. Likewise, there are similar patterns with regard to representation for physicians from Black or Latinx backgrounds: they are much more likely to work in clinical spaces that serve marginalized and resource-deprived patients.

I want to think here about the role of what cultural theorist Kyla Schuller (2017) calls "the biopolitics of feeling" in my conceptualization of affective governance in medical education. Schuller argues: "Bio-power works by situating individuals in dynamic relation and calculating and regulating how their bodies affect one another within a milieu" (2017:11). She claims that affect as a concept links two capacities: those of bodies to form *and* to receive impressions from other bodies. Historically, in the development of science on racial and gendered bodily difference, white women in particular have been constructed as having overly porous bodies, bodies that constantly take in sensations and impressions from the world around them. On the other hand, scholarship on race has portrayed Black people in particular as constantly throwing off impressions and sensations but being incapable of taking these in. Thus, the ability—or lack thereof—to be able to regulate one's capacities for affect is a key aspect of biopolitics that maintains racism. Schuller writes:

> Sentimentalism worked to position the body's differential capacity of feeling as the object and method of state power and capitalist development, a project that works not only through the rehearsal of emotional experience and consumer gratification, but also through the stimulation and regulation of the body's vital capacities (2017:20).

Because white women have been constructed as having this ability to modulate their affects, they have been enfolded into technologies of biopolitics. On the other hand, people of color—in particular, Black and Latinx folks—have been "scientifically" determined to lack these abilities.

What I am trying to articulate here is that affective governance in medical education maps onto population-level dynamics with regard to race and gender. White women are produced by biopolitics as being more amenable to technologies of affect, while white men can hang onto social authority without them. On the other hand, people of color may struggle to embody these forms of social authority precisely because the biopolitics of feeling means that technologies of affect always already exclude them. I see this as a dynamic playing out for both patients and physicians. The normalizing and normative technologies of affect that dictate certain forms of emotional communication read differently depending on the race and gender of their user. Likewise they are shot through with assumptions about the ability to become self-regulating and self-responsible that render some populations compliant and others as in need of more direct forms of disciplinary power.

These technologies of affect in medical education and the health professions are billed as empowering for patients—unshackling them from the physician-centered era of professional dominance—and yet they empower only those patients who are structurally positioned to take up these technologies of the self. They make the exercise of professional dominance more palatable to those with the resources and authority to reject it outright. Moreover, they introduce new emotional demands and technologies on physicians and healthcare providers. In this way, I am not terribly hopeful about a future in which physicians practice mindfulness and patients' inner lives are appreciated without systematic attention being paid to the deeply entrenched structural inequalities produced by capitalism that remain in place in clinical medicine.

This is a very important moment for sociologists, anthropologists, and other critical social scientists concerned with medical education. Our critiques are needed.

Imagining Otherwise: Resistance and Building Structures of Caring

Writing on affective technologies in care work, sociologist Ariel Ducey asks: "How can people be motivated to care—about their jobs, their patients, their employers—when all objective indicators suggest there is little care for them?" (2010:29). Given the seeming omnipresence of affective modes of governance and technologies of affect in contemporary healthcare, how might we reimagine medical education in a landscape where there is very little care for workers or patients? Or where the modes of care are quickly coopted for professional dominance or turned into biovalue to make money for corporatized hospital systems? It seems to me that the current debate about burnout is an opportunity for critiquing the systems that foster alienation and indignity.

I urge for a reimagining of care in structural terms, both in medical education and broadly in healthcare. Discussions about burnout in the medical profession indicate that the structure of work is untenable for many if not most (Shanafelt, Dyrbye, and West 2017; West et al. 2016; West, Dyrbye, and Shanafelt 2018). Certainly, there is a balance to be struck with long work hours for trainees in terms of developing mastery. And yet, the systems that support this kind of long, intense recrafting of the self do not foster care. We urgently need to restructure the physician-patient relationship to allow for longer time with patients, less fragmented care, and better and more mentorship from superiors. However, we also need to reconceptualize the cost, frequency, and stakes of the standardized exams that medical trainees must undergo (Hodges 2006; Patel et al. 2015; Patrício et al. 2013). It would also greatly help alleviate the pressure medical trainees face financially and the elitism of the profession to make medical school more affordable. Too many trainees cannot leave when burned out because of their debt (West, Shanafelt, and Kolars 2011). Medical education could also do more to equip trainees and physicians with the tools to make structural interventions in their patients' lives. Pairing residents with community members to tour neighborhoods and service agencies, for example, helps physicians adopt a structural understanding of health—including the effects of institutional racism (Hansen, Braslow, and Rohrbaugh 2018). Integrating screening tools for structural vulnerability may also foster such awareness (Bourgois et al. 2017). Medical-legal partnerships, in which healthcare teams include lawyers able to address issues such as housing insecurity, have been demonstrated to improve health for marginalized patients (Curran, Paul, and Tobin Tyler 2017; Regenstein et al. 2018; Taylor et al. 2015).

Likewise, patient empowerment should be reconceptualized in medical education and beyond as more than a medical provider's deployment of a set of skills in the encounter. Empowerment without the ability to access resources is meaningless (Braveman et al. 2011; Roberts 2015). The calls to reject and remake institutions of healthcare that feminists and racial justice activists made in the 1960s are still needed today. Patient empowerment requires a *structural* basis. Securing access to healthcare via affordable—perhaps even nationalized—insurance would allow patients the ability to seek preventative healthcare, to get the screenings that could save their lives, to even get the laypeople who make their living playing patients the ability to *be* them. Community-led peer advocacy programs could allow those with access to cultural health capital put theirs to work helping others make demands on physicians (Edmiston 2018).

Finally, medical education must wrestle with structurally embedded racism, sexism, and discrimination against LGBTQAI+ patients. As research demonstrates, knowledge only does so much to reduce unequal treatment—deeply held biases must be changed as well (Stroumsa et al. 2019). It is not enough to put this work onto the Black and Latinx students who make it into medical school despite a structure designed against them (Olsen 2019). To truly empower patients and produce good physicians, medical education must take ownership of the affective economies that circulate in and through it. Partnership with sociologists, anthropologists, and other critical social scientists who have expertise in structures of inequality would be invaluable.

As I write this, there is an exciting resurgence of interest in medical education and the health professions more broadly. Scholars with whom I collaborate and those whose work I admire are doing cutting-edge work to resurrect a field that has not received systemic attention really since the 1960s. And yet it is an area of study that made sociology as a discipline. From these original studies came much of our understandings of professions (Freidson 1988). Furthermore, these early studies involved collaboration between sociologists and medical educators in ways that have fallen by the wayside. But that is changing. With the inclusion of social determinants of health and other sociological topics on the MCAT, medical education is reinvesting in the value of expertise in the social.

This book contributes to this reinvigorated sociology of medical education—indeed, of health professions education—by revisiting classic themes in the professional socialization of medical students with new theoretical tools. In particular, with its emphasis on relationality, bodily impressibility, nonrepresentation, and connectivity, affect theory offers new ways of thinking and understanding clinical work. Likewise, by exploring simulation, I offer new cases for understanding the work of professional socialization.

ACKNOWLEDGMENTS

It is only fitting to include in a book on affect an acknowledgement of all of the forms of care that I received while working on this manuscript.

I am firstly thankful to my participants: the GTAs, medical faculty, and medical students who spent their precious time talking to me. For ten years, I was part of several communities of GTAs. I am very grateful to have known you all. To my friends, coworkers, and fellow activists in reproductive justice: thank you for modeling feminist principles.

At the Department of Sociology at the University of Illinois at Chicago, I was fortunate to work with Claire Laurier Decoteau, Laurie Schaffner, Sandra Sufian, Paul-Brian McInerney, Sydney Halpern, and Lorena Garcia. I started working with Claire my second year of graduate school. I am so grateful for her thoughtful and engaged mentorship, her careful criticism of my work, and the introduction she gave me to theories of the body and biopolitics. Her reading group was one of the foundational experiences of my training. My thanks also to Lisa Berube and Alison Moss for feedback along the way. I received funding from the Alice J. Dan Dissertation Award.

I am grateful to have been a Postdoctoral Research Associate in the Department of Medical Education at the University of Illinois at Chicago. My sincere thanks to Laura Hirshfield, Sandra Sufian (yes, twice!), Ilene Harris, and all my other generous colleagues in that department. Laura has been a fabulous mentor, collaborator, and true friend. I can't thank her enough for providing the material and emotional support that I needed to develop and ultimately finish this book.

I somehow lucked my way into a writing group that provided incisive critique and raucous validation at every step of the way. Jody Ahlm, Danielle Giffort, and Paige L. Sweet are some of the smartest and most generous people around. I thank them for reading endless drafts, hopping on whatever video chat platform we could get to work, and answering texts even when they were just gifs.

My colleagues in the Department of Sociology and the Center for Science, Technology, and Society at Drexel University have been endlessly generous and very smart with their feedback. Thank you to Susan Bell and Kelly Joyce for reading portions of this manuscript and for mentorship along the path to publication. All the gratitude to my cohort of junior colleagues, especially Claire Herbert, Nada Matta, Kevin Moseby, and Jason Orne. My STS colleagues also provided feedback and support, including Alison Kenner and Chloe Silverman.

Ellen Annandale, Laura Mamo, and Stefan Timmermans graciously agreed to read and critique this manuscript in a full-day workshop. I owe them my sincere thanks for traveling so far, reading so closely, and making this book that much stronger.

I owe many thanks to my generous colleagues in the Sociology of Health Professions Education Working Group, in particular: Tania Jenkins, Julia Knopes, Lauren Olsen, and Alexandra Vinson.

Thank you to my colleagues in the United Kingdom who welcomed Susan Bell, Kelly Joyce, and me on a whirlwind intellectual tour. I presented portions of the introduction and Chapter 6 at Cardiff University, University of York, and University of Edinburgh. Their generosity is much appreciated.

I am deeply grateful to everyone at NYU Press: my wonderful editor Ilene Kalish, her assistant Sonia Tsuruoka, and series editors Monica Casper and Lisa Jean Moore. Thank you to Cathy Hannabach at Ideas on Fire for superb developmental editing. Thank you to Diane Judge and the Association of Professors of Gynecology and Obstetrics for allowing me to reprint the materials in the appendices. Portions of chapter 4 were previously published in 2015 as "Playing Doctor: Simulation in Medical School as Affective Practice," *Social Science & Medicine* 136:180–188. Portions of chapter 3 were previously published in 2011 as "'It's the Knowledge that Puts You in Control': The Embodied Labor of Gynecological Educators," *Gender & Society* 25(4):431–450.

My loved ones have sustained me—listened to me, bought me drinks when I needed them, cheered me on. Much love to my fellow writers, Anna Pulley and Katrina Carrasco. Thanks to Becca Cain for the friendship and speedy indexing. My sister, Ana, has been an intellectual champion of mine, maker of wonderful meals, provider of sunny all-seasons rooms, and creator of the absolute best statement necklaces. Thank you.

My mother, Chris, cheered me on and insisted on receiving the first copy of the book. Thanks as well to my grandmother, who doesn't like it when doctors talk down to her because she's old. I love you all. Terri, Paul, and the rest of the Madalinski clan, thanks for welcoming me into your family.

I lost my father, Rik, the summer after my second year of graduate school. I am deeply saddened that he can't see what became of it (and me), but I turned out to be the scholar and person I am because of his love and guidance.

And here, now, gratitude that exists beyond language for one person: my nesting partner, Laura, who has held my hand since the beginning. Thank you for the pep talks when I just couldn't anymore, feeding me when I worked too much, challenging me to make my language more accessible and more intersectional, and just generally sharing your life with me. I love you.

APPENDIX A

Methodology

I worked as a gynecological teaching associate for ten years, starting in 2005 and ending in 2015. I began several years before starting graduate school and continued working as I conducted the research in this book. This raises some interesting questions about methods and knowledge production. As both an insider and outsider, how have I affected and been affected by my subject matter? In a book about emotion and the body, how do my emotions and my body fit into the process of knowledge production?

This question about methodology isn't a new one for feminists. Our core epistemological assumptions attend to the decentering of objectivity as a privileged mode of knowing, even as we strive to find robust methods of assuring that what we know is rigorously grounded in the world. For this reason, I was attracted to Adele Clarke's (2005) postmodernist take on grounded theory called "situational analysis." This is an analytic technique that uses situational maps, social worlds maps, and positional maps to lay out the key actors, discursive positions, and claims of a given phenomenon. However, given my intimate connection to this work, I also found inspiration in feminist work on affect and "research assemblages" (Ringrose and Renold 2014). I had many long conversations with colleagues about that particular quality of qualitative research when you know something in your body because you have experienced it. It is a form, I think, of affective entanglement, as Natasha Myers (2012) has described with regard to molecular biologists.

The Research

The research project that informs this book was multipronged. It included both a historical and a contemporary component, combined interview data with archival data, and situated the phenomenon (teaching and learning the pelvic exam in medical schools) among three key groups of stakeholders. This design perhaps most closely reflects the premises set forth in Clarke's work on situational analysis: I wanted to consider the development and current arrangement of a given social phenomenon. I combined archival sources with interview data in part because of the historical dimension of the work and in part to situate current practices in a national context. I chose three groups of stakeholders (gynecological teaching associates and program coordinators, medical students, and medical faculty) in order to quasi-triangulate the phenomenon. This made for an appropriate way for me to assess the phenomenon from multiple perspectives in order to develop a fuller and more nuanced account of it.

The research proceeded in two stages. First I conducted pilot interviews with GTAs in a variety of cities in the United States in 2009 and 2010. There are no formal networks or professional associations for GTAs, and they are not, strictly speaking, employees of the schools they work for. Consequently, tapping into their informal networks is one of the only ways to connect with them. I suspect that I was able to conduct this research only because of my own participation as a GTA. I circulated a call for participation through some of my current and former coworkers, who passed it along to their networks. These folks vouched for me to their coworkers and friends, which helped with access. If not for my own experience, I doubt I would have known about these programs or how to reach so many GTAs. I had an interesting encounter with my institution's review board at this point. I was not allowed to contact potential participants directly (for example, if Person A said, "Hey, you should talk to Person B. Here is her email address!") because my IRB was concerned that these GTAs might be keeping their job a secret from their families. It seemed as though my IRB was drawing a connection between GTAs and sex work, in a way that stigmatized both. I unpack this in chapter 3. I might have contacted more GTAs if not for this barrier. Instead, I had to wait for them to get in touch with me.

For the second phase of the project, I chose three Chicago-area medical schools to study in depth. I collected archival data and interviewed all three groups of stakeholders between 2011 and 2013. I continued to gather archival data through the completion of the book manuscript in 2019. Again, my insider knowledge shaped the research. Because I worked in Chicago as a GTA, I had a sense of which individual to approach first, which schools had the most well-established program, and what students learned. I used this knowledge to select the schools that I studied. On the other hand, I purposely did not choose any schools where I myself have taught. It might have been a shortcoming, but I could not imagine interviewing a medical student whom I had just taught on my own body. On the other hand, I conducted many interviews with my coworkers, often before we started teaching for the night. In total, I conducted twenty-six interviews with gynecological teaching associates and program coordinators.

My interviews with faculty and staff focused on the pedagogical goals of this type of education and their knowledge of the historical development of the programs. I contacted faculty and staff through medical school websites and asked them to pass along the information sheet for students. I also identified key players in the historical development of these programs, whom I identified through the academic literature. In total, I conducted seven interviews with faculty and staff. My interviews with students focused on the experience of this type of education and how medical students both perceived and interacted with the gynecological teaching associate with whom they worked. There is some evidence as well that students were involved in the push for these programs to be implemented, so I also interviewed former students involved in the early programs. I conducted twenty-three interviews with current and former students. Of the current medical students I interviewed, these were evenly divided by gender.

I also collected over a thousand pages of documentary sources. In order to confirm the historical information that I obtained both from secondary sources and in my interviews, I gathered source materials from medical school archives, archives of the American Association of Medical Colleges, newspapers, and academic journals. Specifically, I was interested in reports published in peer-reviewed journals by medical school faculty on these programs, annual reports and faculty meeting minutes for departments of gynecology, popular newspaper and magazine coverage, and presentations and papers made at AAMC annual meetings. While my focus was specifically on Chicago, I also looked for peer-reviewed articles and reports generated by the AAMC in order to situate Chicago medical schools within broader national debates about these programs. In addition, I was able to gain access to the private collection of one of the originators of GTA programs in Chicago, who had a number of files of handouts, lecture notes, and other development materials in storage.

Gathering materials continued from 2015 to 2017, when I held a postdoctoral position in the Department of Medical Education at the University of Illinois at Chicago, and from 2017 to 2019 when I joined the Department of Sociology at Drexel University. The postdoctoral position was a unique outsider-insider experience that certainly shaped this book project. During that time, I was involved in the behind-the-scenes work of clinical skills education using simulated patients. I debriefed medical students and residents after workshops with simulated patients (both in the classroom and in the simulation center). I sat in on symposiums and discussion groups for medical students. I wrote and revised cases for communication workshops with simulated patients. I attended department meetings and research presentations by leading scholars in medical education research. I presented my own research and had informal conversations with my colleagues about emotional socialization and simulation. I attended medical education research conferences. I collected reports, peer-reviewed articles, meeting minutes, handouts given to the students, and brochures. Those two years indelibly shaped how I have come to understand technologies of affect in medical education.

The Challenges

Doing this kind of research project involved challenges that are standard to any kind of historical and contemporary qualitative study and some that were unique because of my involvement as a GTA. One major limitation is survival in that historical research privileges what is recorded or recalled by participants. I frequently ran into this problem, as many of the sources I wanted to find, such as notes from early feminist meetings, had been lost or destroyed. One of the key innovators of the first Chicagoland GTA program told me that she had destroyed all of her relevant documents just six months before I contacted her. I can only speculate about what might have been in those documents. I was also unable to contact those who had fallen out of touch with their peers or whose names weren't recorded. This was particularly problematic with GTAs. A major player in the first program remains unidentified, as my participants could remember only her first name (a nickname), and no one could remember where she had moved to after leaving Chicago.

Interviewing current and former coworkers required me to be especially attentive to maintaining confidentiality, as my participants would frequently mention one another to me and ask whom I had spoken to and what about. It was impossible to keep them from mentioning doing interviews with me to one another, but I myself did not reveal any of this information. The intimacies of the job bolstered and strained the interviews in interesting ways. Knowing that I also had worked as a GTA may have given some of the GTAs greater freedom in discussing the intimate details of allowing strangers to do such invasive exams on their bodies. However, knowing that I had worked with some of their colleagues may also have encouraged some of them not to engage in more aggressive critiques of one another.

In addition, I was keenly aware that even though I attempted to practice ethical research and minimize power, I still held authority as a researcher. I often found myself in the position of having to explain that I was not yet a doctor and no, I was not going to be that kind of doctor, to the GTAs who did not know me. Even among those who did, my status as a university-affiliated doctoral candidate gave me a certain prestige. One of them in particular liked to ask my opinion on certain practices in the sessions as though I could speak with authority for all of biomedicine. For example, during the research, new guidelines came out about teaching the breast self-exam (BSE). This is a politicized topic for the GTAs I spoke with, since the recommendations to stop teaching the SBE flew in the face of their deeply held beliefs to educate patients about their own bodies and empower them to become comfortable and familiar with their anatomy. This participant in particular asked me my thoughts about these recommendations and to explain why anyone would think this was a good idea.

My interviews with medical faculty and medical students posed a different set of challenges. I went into these interviews on the assumption that this was a clear-cut case of "studying up" since sociology is less prestigious compared to medicine and since at the time I didn't have my PhD. However, perhaps owing to the interdisciplinary nature of medical education departments, the medical faculty I interviewed treated me as a colleague. None of them "talked down" to me when I asked uninformed questions about medical school curricula or medical procedures. Equally, medical students treated me as a colleague, perhaps because I could relate to them about the pressures and trials of graduate education. Gender presented challenges, and sexuality was a constant specter, since I asked detailed questions about the affective experience of intimate exams. At the time, I tended to present as a fairly straight-appearing woman. Men certainly talked to me differently in some ways when I interviewed them face to face as compared with over the phone. For all of the medical students, it seemed that the lesson of desexualizing intimate contact had been deeply imbedded in them. I could practically see the gears turning in medical students' heads about how to discuss a taboo subject honestly—touching a stranger's vagina—without appearing unprofessional. This manifested in a number of pauses, "you know's," and other inferred references to sexuality. For reasons I can't fully explain, I didn't disclose my identity as a GTA to either medical faculty or medical students.

The Analysis

During my interviews, I took detailed notes and used these to begin initial coding and to guide additional interviews. After each interview, I wrote memos to myself to help this process of identifying key themes, discourses, and processes. In this way, I was able to know when I had reached data saturation. I then transcribed all of my interviews or used a transcription service, and I used a combination of open-coding in Word and guided coding in the web-based program Dedoose to track primary and secondary codes and themes. I compared these to the notes and memos I took during the interviews to guide the process. Once I had completed this initial coding, I used situational analysis to analyze my data more fully. As a visual learner and embodied thinker, I found it helpful to sketch out the relationships among people and organizations and/or among concepts and discourses. I also used this technique to develop timelines that tracked key events and key developments in the discourse around GTA programs and medical education reform.

My work was collaborative in that during interviews, I reflected what I thought I was finding back to my participants, and during the analysis process, I asked participants to respond to my findings. I shared drafts of my chapters with several of my GTA participants and invited one of them in particular to attend talks I gave in the Chicagoland area. I then met with her over coffee to talk about her thoughts and impressions on my work. I also shared my work with several of the medical faculty I interviewed to hear their thoughts and impressions. Later, during my postdoctoral work in medical education, I presented my findings and received feedback from leading scholars. This has been an ongoing and interesting aspect of the work, as I have had to learn to translate my critical feminist sociological work into medical-education speak and vice versa.

On Affecting and Being Affected by a Research Topic

Much has been written about how sociologists' positionality shapes our research, and a great deal has also been written about how our research shapes us. From critiques of the notion of objectivity as arising from a privileged social location to concerns over the proliferation of "me-search" to important provocations raised about the line between activism and scholarship, a lot has been said. On the other hand, there is a growing awareness of the ways in which anger can arise when a woman interviews convicted rapists, for example, or the stress and exhaustion that become compounded when persons of color study acts of violence committed against those who share their identities. What I think is interesting is what happens when one is affectively tangled with a research topic, as I was. I must consider how my own affects and the affective intensities that were produced with my research participants shaped this work.

The things-I-knew-but-could-not-name shaped my questions and my analysis. I know at the level of my body what is going on in the pelvic exam. My own embodied memories of the exam shaped how I read and understood accounts of teaching and learning. For example, when I was interviewing one of the medical faculty members, we had a long conversation about the material tinkering (such as learning to angle the fingers down and then up to start the bimanual exam) of the pelvic exam. I couldn't stop thinking about how it has felt to teach on my own body. I could practically feel our conversation in my body, in fact. This in turn shaped the kinds of questions that I asked. Likewise, as I thought through and wrote about the development of embodied habit and experiential knowledge, my own versions of these informed my work. This manifested in a certain amount of "acting out" of the techniques of the pelvic exam and the dispositions of professionalism as I wrote sections attempting to describe these. For example, the only way I have been able to present a discussion of the hand position for the bimanual exam has been to literally act it out during talks. I remain frustrated that the chapter on this does not fully encapsulate the problem. In addition, I continued to work as a GTA during analysis and writing, and I often found myself thinking through problems in my work while I was teaching. Some of my best insights came from hurriedly scribbled memos while I sat in a hospital gown waiting for my next group of students. I have tried my best throughout the manuscript to flag moments where my own affects shaped my analysis.

For a whole array of reasons, I didn't even try to ask my institutional review board to approve observing GTA sessions as part of my research. It would have been fascinating, certainly, but the bureaucratic hurdles would have been enormous: medical schools are extremely protective of outsiders doing research on their students. In addition, the practical concerns were also substantial: the clinic rooms where GTA sessions take place are tiny and my presence would have disrupted the flow of the encounter. I knew this, of course, because of my work as a GTA. This insider knowledge helped me let go of the idea of conducting observations and thus affected the design of this work. As a result, I often found myself using my experience as a practical reference point for my analysis.

Certainly, my insider knowledge of the techniques allowed me to develop rapport with my GTA participants. For example, in chapter 3, I write about the sharing of intimate knowledge in interviews with GTAs, when we would both say "you know" and run out of words to talk about the moment a student locates an ovary. Equally, though, I wonder how my interviews with medical students would have gone had I not been a GTA. Those interviews were also shaped by circulations of affect. Professionalism itself, as I have argued, is a kind of modification of affective states of being. The students I interviewed struggled to discuss matters that violated their newly emerging professional dispositions. For example, as I mentioned in chapters 3 and 4, I had challenges trying to get my interviewees to talk about sexuality. I remember one interview with a man who was doing everything he could to *not* say that the exam wasn't a problem for him because he found the GTAs unattractive. It was one of those moments when I couldn't figure out how to ask a question to check that the thing I was feeling was really happening. To have asked outright would have horrified him, so I tried various forms of the same question until we both understood that the other person knew what we were trying to do. This happened during an in-person interview. It's challenging to get medical students to participate in half-hour interviews, even though I offered to meet students wherever was convenient for them. Hence, I offered the phone as an option and conducted about half of the interviews that way. (I didn't know anyone doing interviews over Skype, so I didn't consider it.) The introduction of the material object of the phone into the research-assemblage likely shifted the kinds of connection I could make with the medical students I interviewed.

In all of these ways, I have attended to the flows of affect that have animated the research process for me. My experience with the subject matter, my own embodied identity, and my interests and political commitments have most certainly shaped the text.

APPENDIX B

Pelvic Exam Checklists

Gynecology Clerkship
Pelvic Examination Instruction
Developed by Ms. Reiter, Ms. Hamilton,
and Ms. Guenther

130

DESCRIPTION AND GUIDE FOR CONDUCTING A QUALITY PELVIC EXAMINATION

I. Facilitating Patient Comfort, Cooperation, and Relaxation

The interaction during a pelvic examination can be divided into those behaviors which are solely the responsibility of the doctor, including verbal and nonverbal behavior, and those which require active participation of the patient, patient's cooperative behavior. Attention to all three types of interaction sets a climate to facilitate a quality pelvic exam.

Doctor's Verbal Behavior

1. Acknowledge patient's anxiety (i.e., "You seem nervous about this exam, and that's understandable.").

2. Inquire if she has had difficulty with previous pelvic exams.

3. Assure her that you will do your best to make the exam comfortable.

4. Provide patient with rationale for need to relax.

5. Assure patient all procedures and instructions will be shown and explained.

6. Give patient permission to stop you if exam is uncomfortable.

7. Elicit verbal commitment from patient.

8. Ask if patient is as physically comfortable as possible before proceeding with exam.

9. Use appropriate level of terminology, i.e., "not too scientific and not too condescending".

10. Avoid vocabulary with sexual connotations.

11. Avoid inappropriate humor.

12. Use supportive tone of voice.

Doctor's Nonverbal Behavior

1. Check patient is physically comfortable before and during exam.

2. Give verbal cues before physical cues.

3. Equalize power space as soon as possible.

4. Protect patient's personal space.

5. Use slow motions which allow patient to maintain relaxation.

6. Avoid unnecessary physical contact and pressure.

7. Remember to exert posterior pressure.

8. Avoid undue familiarity.

9. Maintain eye contact with patient.

10. Use lubricant generously.

11. Drape patient to facilitate eye contact and patient monitoring.

Figure B.1a–e. From "Description and Guide for Conducting a Quality Pelvic Examination," Ms. Reiter, Ms. Hamilton, and Ms. Guenther.

Patient's Cooperative Behavior

131

1. Patient agrees to have head raised, which relaxes muscles and places her in a more equal position.

2. Patient agrees to become involved in exam, i.e. feeling her own uterus, nodes, or holding sheet.

3. Patient agrees to lift gown, which gives her control of exposing her body.

4. Patient becomes aware of tense muscles and learns to relax them.

5. Patient learns to control breathing, i.e. "take a deep breath".

6. Patient learns to relax her knees out to the side, i.e. "let your knees fall out to my hands".

7. Patient supports her thighs when necessary.

II. Abdominal Exam

The abdominal exam provides an opportunity to build a sense of trust and rapport with the patient which makes a quality pelvic exam possible. Attention to certain interpersonal factors is useful for this purpose, recognizing that even a healthy patient has a certain amount of anxiety which interferes with her cooperation. It is therefore necessary to allow the patient time to cooperate with your verbal requests. It is also useful to slow down your physical motions in order to allow her time to maintain the required muscular relaxation, to monitor your patient's tenseness and to use relaxation technique. Whenever possible, use verbal instructions and allow patient to move her own body.

1. Inform patient exam is about to begin.

2. Assist with positioning patient, i.e. remember to extend shelf.

3. Ask for patient's assistance if necessary.

4. Ask if there is any tenderness.

5. Invite patient to inform of any discomfort.

6. Inform patient of superficial and/or deep palpation.

7. Use warm hands.

8. Explain exam as you proceed, i.e., "I am checking your liver", etc.

9. Examine four quadrants.

10. Feel for masses.

11. Feel for liver, spleen, lymph nodes, pulses.

12. Observe and comment on abnormalities (scars).

III. Positioning and Preparing Patient for Pelvic Exam

The transfer from the abdominal exam to the pelvic exam is typically a time of increased anxiety for the patient. The doctor can help alleviate much of this anxiety by maintaining contact with the patient while she is being positioned and by attending to certain of her physical requirements.

1. Inquire if patient is ready (transition phase).

2. Introduce the nurse and ask her/him to assist.

Figure B.1a–e. (*continued*)

-3-   132

3. Raise the back of the exam table.

4. Assist her feet into stirrups.

5. Assist with the pillow.

6. Assist the patient to slide down to the level of a hand placed at end of table.

7. See that drapes are correctly arranged to facilitate eye contact--i.e. "I can see you / you can see me."

8. Ask if patient is comfortable.

9. Ask about previous experiences and offer reassurance where necessary.

10. Sit down as soon as possible to equalize space.

IV. Exam of External Genitalia

There are two important principles to remember during examination of the external genitalia: first, the patient is practically blind in the lithotomy position and needs to be given verbal descriptions of all your actions; second, preventive medicine requires a degree of comfort with looking at genitals sufficient to allow careful visual investigation of the external genitalia.

1. Enlist patient's cooperation and request. Wait, i.e. "let knees fall out to my hands".

2. Wait for patient's cooperation--recognize anxiety interrupts that cooperation.

3. Verbal cue followed by tactile cue--hand on thigh.

4. Hand on outside of vagina. "Now I am going to touch the outside of your vagina."

5. Hand on labia. "Now I am going to be spreading your labia."

6. Include these structures: clitoris, Bartholin glands, Skene's glands, periurethral glands, and the introitus.

7. Use smooth versus jabbing motion of fingers.

V. Speculum Exam, Papanicolaou Smear, and GC Culture

Since for the majority of patients it is neither possible nor advisable to attempt to distract her from the necessary interference with her physical integrity (the patient's fantasy of distress can be far worse than the reality), it is advisable to allay anticipatory anxiety by a thorough explanation and display of all instruments and procedures and to contract with the patient to stop and make adjustments if any part of the exam is creating distress. Physicians have the responsibility to inform their patients of the meaning and importance of regularly making appointments for cancer and VD screening tests.

1. Select correct sized speculum. If not, change.

2. Show and explain speculum.

3. Tell patient, "The speculum might feel cool."

4. Spread labia and introitus to create opening.

5. Use posterior pressure, inserting downward and inward.

6. Check for resistance from dryness or pubic hair.

7. Verbalize--"Some women have discomfort and some don't--let me know if you are uncomfortable."

Figure B.1a–e. (*continued*)

-4-   133

8. Pass Ayers spatula, cotton swab, and any other instruments in patient's line of vision.

9. Explain that the Papanicolaou smear is a cancer detection test.
   a. Collect cells with Ayers spatula. (Ayers spatula--rotated, spread out thinly on slide, and fixed.)
   b. Insert cotton tip into os. (Cotton swab--rotated, rolled on slide, and fixed.)
   c. Obtain GC culture--explain that this is routine for all patients.

10. Remove speculum.
    a. Lift blades off cervix.
    b. Remember--posterior pressure.
    c. Rotate speculum--tell patient.
    d. Visual exam--progressive observation.

VI. Bimanual Exam

A relaxed, comfortable patient is essential in order to palpate her internal structures. It is helpful to involve your patient by eliciting her cooperation and active participation in relaxing the abdominal muscles. Monitor your patient's face for cues as to her comfort. Also, it is useful to monitor the patient for muscle tension. If she seems to be resisting, it helps to slow down to give her a chance to work with you instead of against you.

1. Use lubricating jelly generously on hairs, labia, backs of gloved fingers, and introitus.

2. Apply downward pressure at fourchette.

3. Pause to enhance relaxation.

4. Insert middle and forefinger into vagina.

5. Position your body for proper angle and strength.

6. Inform patient she will be feeling firm pressure and possibly some tenderness.

7. Check muscle relaxation--if not present, give patient specific instructions about how to relax, i.e. deep breaths, paying attention to muscle tension.

8. Involve the patient in exam, i.e., describe cervix, offer her the option to feel uterus.

9. Palpate the cervix, noting:
   a. Size.
   b. Position.
   c. Contour.
   d. Consistency.
   e. Movement of the cervix. Stretch uterosacral and transverse cervical ligaments.
   f. Mobility.
   g. Pelvic tenderness.
   h. Appropriate pressure.
   Give description of this procedure and findings to the patient during the examination.

10. Palpate the uterus, noting:
    a. Position.
    b. Size.
    c. Mobility.
    d. Tenderness.
    e. Contour.

Figure B.1a–e. (*continued*)

134

f. Consistency.
g. Appropriate pressure.
Give description of this procedure and findings to the patient during the examination.

11. Palpate the ovaries, noting:
    a. Right.
    b. Left.
    c. Appropriate pressure.
    d. Facial observation of patient.

12. Apply pressure while patient exhales.

VII. Rectovaginal Exam

A quality pelvic exam is not complete without a confirmatory rectovaginal exam. This part of the exam need not be uncomfortable if you wait for the sphincter muscle to relax, use slow motions, and give the patient verbal support.

1. Inform patient verbally, i.e., "I will be inserting one finger in your rectal sphincter and one finger in your vagina."

2. Relubricate rectal finger.

3. Instruct patient to relax anal sphincter, i.e., "Bear down against my finger."

4. Insert rectal finger anteriorly until through anal sphincter then angle posteriorly.

5. Examine septum between two fingers.

6. "Reach up" with extended rectal finger past cervix to examine cul-de-sac, uterosacral and sacrococcygeal ligaments.

7. Palpate to confirm vaginal findings of cervix, uterus (posterior aspect), and ovaries.

VIII. Closure of the Exam

Often since a patient will wait until the last minute to voice any concerns, it is important at this point to offer an opportunity for her to ask questions.

1. Assist patient to sit up out of the lithotomy position immediately.

2. Summarize and discuss exam findings with patient.

3. Indicate how patient will receive lab reports.

4. Elicit and respond to any patient questions.

Figure B.1a–e. (*continued*)

Pelvic Examination Checklist – Observation of Clinical Skills

Checklists may be used for teaching and/or for assessment. Grading may be by yes/no or expanded to include assessment of task completion to fully/partially/not done/not applicable.

The checklist should be completed by a trained observer with knowledge of the proper technique of the pelvic examination. Due to the nature of the techniques required, an in-room observer is the minimum essential. In addition, the checklist may be completed by a trained remote (video) observer (useful for assessment of communication and interpersonal skills while the in-room observer focuses on technical skills) and/or the patient or model/GTA.

Student: _____   Date: _____   Evaluator: _____

Direct Observation of the Patient	Well Done	Needs Improvement	Not Done	Cannot Recall
Communication/Interpersonal Skills				
Introduces self and explains role				
Establishes names/relationships of family				
Starts with an open-ended question				
Uses appropriate eye contact, body language				
Uses facilitative listening skills				
Demonstrates empathy				
Preparation				
Checks all equipment/supplies				
Adjusts exam light prior to gloving				
Washes hands				
General Techniques/Exam Skills				
Demonstrates concern for the patient's comfort and modesty				
Explains to patient/parent what is being done				
Enlists the patient's/parent's cooperation during the exam				
Follows a logical sequence of exam from one region to another				
Emphasizes areas of importance as suggested by interview				

11

Figure B.2a–c. From "The Pelvic Exam," Association of Professors of Gynecology and Obstetrics.

Modifies the exam to adapt to patient limitations (imposed by illness, age or temperament of patient)				
Positions patient on back, hips to end of table and heels on foot rests				
Wears gloves throughout exam				
Gloves remain clean (no contamination)				
Avoids unexpected/sudden movements				
External Examination				
Examines external genitalia				
Inspects mons pubis				
Inspects labia majora				
Inspects labia minora				
Inspects clitoris				
Inspects urethal meatus				
Inspects introitus				
Inspects Bartholin's gland				
Inspects perineum				
Inspects anus				
Speculum Examination				
Holds speculum at 45-degree angle				
Inserts speculum properly				
Rotates speculum at full insertion				
Opens speculum slowly				
Identifies cervix				
Secures speculum in open position				
Inspects cervix				
Inspects vaginal walls while removing speculum				
Handles speculum appropriately				
Removes speculum appropriately				
Bimanual Pelvic Examination				
Introduces fingers into vagina				
Palpates cervix and cervical os				
Palpates uterine body, apex of fundus				
Notes uterine size				
Describes position of uterus				
Palpates right adnexa/ovary				

12

Figure B.2a–c. (*continued*)

Palpates left adnexa/ovary				
Bimanual Rectovaginal (RV) Examination				
Re-gloves for RV exam				
Asks patient to bear down as finger is inserted				
Inserts middle finger into rectum				
Inserts index finger into vagina				
Palpates uterus				
Palpates right adnexa/ovary				
Palpates left adnexa-ovary				
Removes fingers smoothly				
Professional Conduct/Additional Skills				
Describes each step of exam to patient prior to performing				
Maintains patient modesty				
Attends to patient's comfort				
Performed exam in a gentle and professional manner				
Extends bottom of exam table for patient comfort				
Instructs patient to return to sitting position at conclusion of exam				
Patient Education Skills (when appropriate)				
Elicits patient's understanding of problem				
Addresses beliefs, misconceptions				
Gives explanations in clear language, avoids jargon				
Invites questions/checks for understanding				

SUMMARY OF OBSERVATION: (Please include assessment of performance and areas of future focus)

FEEDBACK GIVEN: ___YES   ___NO

OVERALL GRADE: Below Expected Level   At Expected Level   Above Expected Level

FACULTY SIGNATURE:_____**STUDENT SIGNATURE:**_____

13

Figure B.2a–c. (*continued*)

NOTES

INTRODUCTION

1 I am not suggesting that feelings between physicians and patients are new or have never mattered, but that the expert apparatus around feelings is new. For examples of how physicians related to patients prior to the rise of scientific medicine in the nineteenth century, see Jewson (1976) on bedside medicine.

2 The pelvic exam has long been of fascination for sociologists, as a space in which one person willingly submits their naked, vulnerable body and its interiors to another person, usually a woman to a man, in a way that both parties attempt to desexualize (Emerson 1970; Henslin and Biggs 1971; Smith and Kleinman 1989). In this space, the rules, it seems, of social reality fall apart.

3 This controversial practice still occurs in medical schools today (Friesen 2018). In such an encounter, novice trainees do pelvic exams on the unconscious bodies of patients who have not given their explicit consent. Often, they are not even told afterward that the exam took place.

4 I use the umbrella term of "simulated patient" as opposed to the more specific term of "standardized patient" through this book. A simulated patient is any layperson who roleplays for the purposes of education or evaluation. Standardized patients are carefully trained in order to evaluate students. For more on this distinction, see Epstein (2007).

5 Throughout the book, I use gender-neutral language to describe those who may have pelvic exams. There are times, however, when I default to using the term "woman" to describe these patients, and in the interest of specificity, I mean cisgender women. It is important to point out that not all women have uteruses, cervixes, and vaginas, and not all people who have this anatomy are women. This book deals almost exclusively with the issue of the pelvic exam for cisgender women, but there is an important conversation about pelvic exams for transgender men and genderqueer or gender nonconforming folks to be had elsewhere.

6 Annie Sprinkle is an artist, educator, activist, and former sex worker with a PhD in Human Sexuality. In the early 1990s, she put on a performance art piece called "Public Cervix Announcement" in which she inserted a speculum in herself and invited members of the audience to come view her cervix. Images of her performance show her reclining calmly in an elaborate chair with a speculum inserted into her vagina while different people point flashlights and peer curiously down its bills.

7 The theory of professional dominance emerged from the work of sociologists Eliot Freidson (1984, 1988) and Paul Starr (1982). According to Starr, in the nineteenth and early twentieth centuries, the cultural authority of the physician reshaped patients' experiences such that the physician became the intermediary between science and the patient: "Once people began to regard science as a superior and legitimately complex way of explaining and controlling reality, they wanted physicians' interpretations of experience regardless of whether the doctors had remedies to offer" (Starr 1982:19). Thus, the professional interests of physicians were served by control over these scientific explanations.

8 In the United States, prior to the late eighteenth and early nineteenth centuries, physicians learned to practice medicine through apprenticeships, by traveling to universities in Europe, or through informal means (Rothstein 1987). There was no legislation that prohibited who could practice medicine, as we have today through licensing and accreditation. During the first half of the nineteenth century, medical schools were often run by a group of four to eight physicians, who trained enrollees as a money-making endeavor (Rothstein 1987). The result was a growing number of poorly trained physicians and a patchwork of medical schools and other adjacent traineeship schools. This changed in the late nineteenth century, as the profession of medicine began to shore up its authority in order to increase its control over the public's trust and access to science.

9 These governing bodies were successful in reducing the number of medical schools. As Rothstein (1987) and others have noted, the schools that closed were more often those that served women and/or people of color. This led to the homogenous medical student body that formed in the early twentieth century: white upper- or middle-class men.

10 Critic and reformer of US higher education, Abraham Flexner, published his eponymous report in 1910. Flexner proposed dividing the four years of medical school into two years of basic sciences and two years of clinical sciences. Subsequently, many medical schools increased the number and rigor of their basic science courses and began to use hospital for training in the clinical sciences.

11 In the 1970s and 1980s, as these changes to the profession occurred, scholars debated whether what had happened was deprofessionalization, proletariatization, or something else (Freidson 1984; Haug 1988; Light 1991; McKinlay and Arches 1985). Sociologist Donald Light (1991) described these forces as "countervailing powers."

12 Part of the increasing stringency of medical licensing was the concern about International Medical Graduates (IMGs), which continues today. These are physicians who have been trained abroad—either in their home country or in places like the Caribbean, where there is what amounts to a cottage industry for educating students who could not get into an MD or DO program in the United States. See Jenkins (2018).

13 The USMLE is currently divided into three parts or "steps" taken at different moments during medical training. Step 1 is typically taken at the end of the second

year and covers basic sciences information. Step 2 is typically taken at the end of the third year and involves clinical knowledge and skills. The more controversial half of Step 2 is the clinical skills (CS) portion, during which medical students must interact with a standardized patient who typically presents a chief compliant (headache, chest pain, and so on). The standardized patient then evaluates the student's performance on skills such as using nontechnical language, showing concern, and sharing their findings and treatment plan. Step 3 is typically taken after the first year of residency and covers more advanced medical knowledge.

14 This movement came as medical faculty began to reconsider and reject the Flexnerian model (Finnerty et al. 2010; Irby, Cooke, and O'Brien 2010; Mann 2011). As a result, basic and clinical sciences were increasingly integrated with courses on professionalism. For more on professionalism see Hafferty and Castellani (2011).

15 Many hospitals and insurance companies now offer online portals allowing patients to view their coverage for specific providers and tests or procedures. Patients are encouraged to take charge of their healthcare costs by seeking out the most affordable option. And yet cost of care is not the only determining factor. A variety of websites, many of them linked to patient portals, now report patient satisfaction and reviews of providers. Patients can rate their interaction with providers and leave comments about their experiences. Hospitals and clinics routinely ask patients to provide satisfaction metrics, which are tied into insurance reimbursement (Fenton et al. 2012; Kupfer and Bond 2012). A physician who is well-liked by patients in these metrics may receive an annual bonus or other financial incentive.

16 Attention to affect as part of a broader program in new materialisms has had broad-reaching effects on a variety of fields of study (Coole and Frost 2010; Devellennes and Dillet 2018; Pitts-Taylor 2016). At the same time, in sociology, there has been a resurgence of interest in emotion (Bonilla-Silva 2018). These scholarly pursuits are responding to and perhaps heightened by interlocking sets of national and global political crises. Questions about the exercise of power in this new economic and political order have prompted new theories of social life, and new materialist theories in particular respond to the limits of representation (i.e., discourse) to explain enduring inequalities and new types of capital (Pitts-Taylor 2016).

17 Deleuze and Guattari think of affect as a pre-personal vital force that animates bodily becomings. They argue, following Spinoza: "We know nothing about a body until we know what it can do, in other words, what its affects are, how they can or cannot enter into composition with other affects, with the affects of another body, either to destroy that body or to be destroyed by it, either to exchange actions and passions with it or to join with it in composing a more powerful body" (1987: 257).

18 Studies demonstrate that in emergency departments, Black children receive substantially less pain medicine when they present the same symptoms of ap-

pendicitis as white children (Goyal et al. 2015). Affect more thoroughly captures the circulations of fear, hostility, and degradation that arise from historical and contemporary racism.

19 The target of control is not making subjects who behave in socially appropriate ways, but "a never-ending modulation of moods, capacities, affects, and potentialities, assembled in genetic codes, identification numbers, ratings profiles, and preference listings . . . in bodies of data and information" (Clough et al. 2007:19). For more on how affect is used to control and direct populations, see also Jackie Orr's (2006) work on psychopolitics.

20 For a very brief overview of a complicated literature, see Blanch-Hartigan 2012; Blanch-Hartigan, Andrzejewski, and Hill 2012; Blanch-Hartigan and Ruben 2013; DiMatteo et al. 1980; DiMatteo, Hays, and Prince 1986; Hall, Andrzejewski, and Yopchick 2009.

21 See also Eva Illouz's (2007) work on emotional capitalism.

22 There has been recent attention in sociology and science studies to the role of emotion in expert work (Craciun 2018; Daston 1995; Myers 2012; Timmermans 2011). These studies analyze how emotion gets leveraged as a tool in expert work and a resource for legitimating expert knowledge claims.

23 I draw this phrase from a growing body of work on "governing with feeling" (Jupp, Pykett, and Smith 2016), which considers how contemporary modes of state, civil, and medical logics for guiding the conduct of the population increasingly operate through emotions, feelings, and affective capacities (Anderson 2012; Barrios 2017; Brown 2015; Clough 2003; Orr 2006; Richard and Rudnyckyj 2009). The phrase "affective governance" comes from the work of geographers Eleanor Jupp, Jessica Pykett, and Fiona M. Smith to capture "the work involved in *governing the emotional states* of citizens" and "*emotional forms of governance*" (2016:3, emphasis original). This theorization of affective governance, as well as the work of sociologist Patricia T. Clough on affect and control, are deeply feminist in their origins, in that they are interested in denaturalizing the biological body, and with it emotion, and are committed to understanding how "feminized" labor is central to new projects of state and expert rule. These forms of governance emerge in conditions of late modern capitalism and the fragmentation of institutions of civic society. Cultural theorist Sara Ahmed (2004, 2015) also brings a feminist perspective to bear in her analysis of the work that emotions do in circulation has been central to the "affective turn." Work on affective governance has come primarily from anthropologists and geographers, but it is an extremely useful concept for sociologists.

CHAPTER 1. THE PELVIC EXAM AND THE POLITICS OF CARE

1 I use first names in this book for all participants interviewed. Since part of my argument is about the ways in which expertise and feminist politics are mutually articulated, my using first names also challenges hierarchies of authority in biomedicine that are reinforced by titles. I use description instead to indicate

who has a PhD or MD. All names provided are pseudonyms, with one exception. Charles R. B. Beckmann is the only real name I use in this book, which I do with permission. I use Charles instead of the name he goes by socially (RB) to align with my pseudonym practices in the book.

2 In his history of medical knowledge, Foucault claims that the body has been transformed into a knowable object and disease into a constellation of signs and symptoms through the development of clinical practice. Foucault uses the term "medical gaze" to refer to the way in which biomedicine (and individual physicians) observes the body: "the gaze that sees is the gaze that dominates" (1994:39).

3 Scholars working in a Deleuzian tradition use the term "assemblage" to understand how heterogeneous, transportable objects and signs are brought together together in practice (Bell 2019; DeLanda 2019; Deleuze and Guattari 1987; Lakoff 2017; Murphy 2012; Ong and Collier 2008; Thompson 2005). Deleuze and Guattari describe assemblages as being semiotic, material, and social, and identifiable by their rhizomatic connection. Deleuze and Guattari take the metaphor of the rhizome from the root structure of some plants, which shoot out in all directions rather than following a linear progression: "A rhizome ceaselessly establishes connections between semiotic chains, organizations of power, and circumstances relative to the arts, sciences, and social struggles" (Deleuze and Guattari 1987:7). Rhizomes defy analyses that insist on origins, and their elements are constantly deterritorializing and reterritorializing, meaning that they hang together (and become institutionalized, for example) and fall apart in ungeneralizable ways.

4 Maria Puig de la Bellacasa writes: "Understanding caring as something we do extends a vision of care as an ethically and politically charged *practice*, one that has been at the forefront of feminist concern with devalued labor" (2011:90, emphasis original). Likewise, work on the "materialities of care" (Buse, Martin, and Nettleton 2018) extends this notion of care as both practice and material engagement. In a special issue of *Sociology of Health and Illness,* Christina Buse, Daryl Martin, and Sarah Nettleton argue that materialities of care "provide a novel way in to examining 'practices of care' as they unfold in a range of formal and informal settings, and in relational ways, whereby embodied, routine and often unnoticed actions of caring are constituted through and between the relations between bodies, objects and spaces" (2018:245). These theorizations of care as an affective or emotionally charged doing in the world are what I draw from as I think of care and caring practices and relationships.

5 Such forcible examinations have always been a routine part of state surveillance of sex workers. Up until the 1960s, the US government arrested sex workers (or simply women accused of sex work), forced them to undergo pelvic exams, and jailed them as part of the "American Plan" to tackle sexually transmitted infections (Stern 2018).

6 As historian Deirdre Cooper Owens (2017) argues in her history of the racist origins of American gynecology, Sims and his contemporaries' development of

reproductive medicine on the bodies of enslaved Black women both extracted further reproductive labor from them and extracted professional capital for their nascent field of study. As part of a more widespread effort to rethink Sims's legacy, his statue in Central Park was removed in 2018. For more on race, exploitation, and the history of gynecology, see Washington (2006), McGregor (1998), Snorton (2017), and Kapsalis (1997).

7　These women go unnamed in the records. On the politics of this, see Snorton (2017) and Kuppers (2008).

8　For more on the normalizing power of reproductive healthcare, see Mamo (2007).

9　By the mid-1950s, in thirty-seven states, couples who applied for a wedding license had to be examined for sexually transmitted infections; for women, this usually meant a pelvic exam (Kavinoky 1954; Lewis 2005).

10　Weiss (1975:24–25) also reports that this textbook (*Obstetrics and Gynecology*) recommends surgery on an unperforated hymen causing pain during intercourse *without* anesthesia for "the purpose of 'demonstrating to the patient that she is quite capable of withstanding the discomfort. . . . Pain . . . is usually a valuable part of therapy.'"

11　Susan Bell provides a fascinating example of how women could sometimes resist these practices in her discussion of Esther's pelvic exam (2009:104–110). In this narrative, Esther, resists the construction of her body as an object of medical knowledge while her physician shows off the vagina he has fashioned for her to groups of medical students by gently teasing him about the practice.

12　See Murphy (2012, 2015) on protocol feminism.

13　Terri Kapsalis (1997) argues that the hiring of sex workers reinforced the construction of the pelvic exam as a sexual rite of passage: an older uncle-figure in the form of the experienced physician hires a sex worker so that his nervous, inexperienced protégé can become a man. What the sex worker herself desires or what her knowledge and expertise provides is omitted by the boy-to-man narrative.

14　Prior to the development of simulated patients, medical students practiced their physical exam skills primarily on clinic patients (Prentice 2013), on a limited number of manikins (Buck 1991), and on themselves (Harris 2016). The advent of human-based simulation in the 1960s was a radically new educational form for medical trainees, and the complexity of manikin-based simulation has only accelerated alongside it.

15　Elizabeth Fee (1975) has drawn distinctions between strands of feminism by using the language of liberal and radical feminism. Under this topology, liberal feminists see the promise of change being possible within existing institutions, whereas radical feminists see change being possible only by outright rejecting existing institutions. There are of course a lot of nuances in feminist theory around these issues, but this highlights the variety of activist stances toward the institutions that they protest (Epstein 2008; Goldner 2004).

16 Another school that I studied in Chicago also created a GTA program because of the demands of a woman medical student. At this school, however, the
pathway came not through a feminist self-help clinic but through the school's
nurse midwifery program. The medical school responded to the student's
demands by recruiting a nurse midwife to teach the pelvic exam to the medical
students. She incorporated principles from nursing that were very similar to
those at the Emma Goldman Health Center and recruited women to work as
GTAs.

17 These feminist challenges were part of a broader organized protest as patients
increasingly began to choose alternatives to mainstream biomedicine for their
reproductive healthcare. Such endeavors offered a direct material challenge to
biomedicine by undermining its economic control. The growth of feminist self-
help clinics took money away from physicians when a critical mass of women
began to use them instead. "Women were recognized as a major health market
in the early 1980s" (Thomas and Zimmerman 2007:364). As more women fled
biomedicine for feminist alternatives, hospitals began to develop "women's health
centers." These centers used the language and practices developed within feminist
spaces to win back their customers.

18 While the focus of this chapter is on the development of the program at UIC,
this aspect can be seen elsewhere as well. Martha, who created a GTA program at
another medical school in Chicago and who used to give a lecture to the medical
students before they went into the session, told me, "Nobody ever talked to the
medical students about, you know, gosh, you may have feelings about cutting
up a cadaver. . . . You're what, twenty-one, twenty-two, you may have feelings
about doing a pelvic exam on a woman because it was mostly male students at
the time. . . . One of the things that I addressed was their feelings about doing
this type of exam, what fears they might have, embarrassment, fear of becoming aroused, touching a woman in this particular way. And then how women felt
about having the exam, which is another thing that was not discussed in medical
school at that time."

19 Most guidelines also suggest that Pap smears not be collected while the patient is
menstruating, as the endometrial cells may interfere with the results. This means
that in actuality, most physicians will not be performing a "well-woman" exam on
a menstruating person.

20 Two coordinators working at this time in two separate GTA programs told me
that they had learned not to hire anyone into the program who espoused an
explicitly feminist agenda. Martha told me, "I was recruiting from the feminist
community, which turned out not to be a good idea. . . . They would come with an
agenda and that wasn't the point. The point was to teach medical students how to
do good exams. They didn't need a lecture about the feminist agenda. Fine, I agree
with your politics, but that's not what you need to be doing."

21 Certainly, the Women's Health Movement wasn't alone in being defanged by con-
servative forces that arose during the Reagan era in the United States (and under

neoliberalism more globally): other rights-based movements—Black Power, queer liberation, student protest—all either simply lost momentum or were actively tamped down by government actions during the 1980s (Freeman and Johnson 1999).

CHAPTER 2. FROM ASSESSING KNOWLEDGE TO ASSESSING PERFORMANCE

1 "Pelvic Exam Instruction" was provided to me by one of my participants out of this individual's personal files. My participant and I made every effort to locate its authors, but were unsuccessful. Despite its unknown (and unaccredited) origins, this document is still circulated among GTAs in Chicago.

2 While I was working as a GTA in Chicago, we used this form or a very similar one to systematically rate a student's performance on all components of the exam. My interviews with GTAs across the United States confirm that this is routine practice—nearly every GTA with whom I spoke said they have to do this. The form then gets labeled with the student's name and submitted to the director of the professionalism course during which the student encounters a GTA.

3 Prior to the 1980s, a typical medical student in the United States was unlikely to have any interactions with patients that were observed in a systematic fashion. In fact, prior to the 1970s, even efforts to teach medical students how to interact with patients were limited in the formal curriculum. It was assumed that a medical student's "bedside manner" could be honed by observing senior physicians and developing his (and I use the masculine deliberately) own style as he gained more experience. Becoming an expert meant mastering scientific knowledge about the human body. When students were tested by their schools or for a national licensing exam, it was this knowledge that exams covered, whether through a written, oral, or practical (bedside) modality.

4 There has been a wealth of research on the use of checklists in medicine, especially in terms of surgical safety checklists (Bosk et al. 2009). There has also been a great deal of research on clinical practice guidelines and evidence-based medicine (Timmermans and Berg 1997, 2010). Less attention has been paid to communication and interpersonal checklists, guidelines, and inventories. What these have in common with other studies of standards and standard-setting in clinical medicine is a flattening out of complex realities via tick-box exercises, on the ground tinkering to make standards "work," resistance over concerns about professional jurisdiction, and the production of new skillsets alongside the diminishing of older ones. I find the communication and interpersonal skills checklist different than some others in that the *object* of control in the checklist is much fuzzier. Surgical checklists, for example, target patient *outcomes*—the patient lives or dies. The object of control of the communication and interpersonal skills checklist is standardizing physician behavior to produce greater patient satisfaction and compliance.

5 Medical expertise is a set of knowledges and practices about the pursuit and maintenance of health and the treatment or management of disease. "Medical expertise, as distinct from medical doctors, is strengthened by letting patients take part in decisions about the direction of research and the aims of medical intervention, that is, by allowing the demand for medical expertise to be coproduced" (Eyal 2013:876). Thus defined, it is most clearly the domain of physicians, but it expands to encompass other healthcare professionals and, importantly, patients.

6 Medical education research as a distinct discipline is interesting to situate alongside the general trend in medicine toward standardization and scientization, as it represents these trends while also being haunted by their limits. Medical education research is a field oriented primarily to objective, scientific knowledge production. And yet, because the work of physicians deals intimately with human suffering and death, medical education as a discipline must also be adaptive to the social and, more specifically, emotional.

7 In 1953, the American Association of Medical Colleges (AAMC) formed a Committee on Teaching Institutes and Special Studies (Kuper, Albert, and Hodges 2010). By 1957 this committee had been renamed the Committee on Research and Education and oversaw efforts to study changes to the curriculum such as the comprehensive medicine programs that I described above. In 1958 in London, the very first medical education research conference was held, called the Association for the Study of Medical Education (Kuper, Albert, and Hodges 2010). The *Journal of Medical Education* (now *Academic Medicine*) published these conference proceedings in 1959. Many of these projects were funded by the Kellogg Foundation and the Commonwealth Fund.

8 While the AAMC had been publishing the premier *Journal of Medical Education* (now titled *Academic Medicine*) since 1926, other specialized journals began to appear. One of the flagship journals, *Medical Education*, published its first issue in 1967. Another key journal, *Medical Teacher*, started publishing in 1979.

9 Sociologist Eva Illouz makes a similar argument about the incorporation of psychology into corporate management styles: "Emotional capitalism is a culture in which emotional and economic discourses and practices mutually shape each other" (2007:5). She traces the rise of communication skills in corporate management as "a new object of knowledge which in turns generates new instruments and practices of knowledge" (2007:18).

10 This is not unlike some current concerns about USMLE step 2 CS (discussed in chapter 6).

11 The data that I present in this chapter are also confirmed by informational interviews that I conducted with leaders in the Department of Medical Education at UIC as part of my research.

12 For more on the current state of master's and PhD programs in Health Professions Education, see Tekian (2014) and Tekian and Harris (2012).

13 For the difference between simulated and standardized patients, see Epstein (2007).

14 They offered no explanation in their published work of what criteria were used to assess who was considered an expert.

15 Other studies such as Kretzschmar's work (1978) and a report from Harvard Medical School on the Pelvic Teaching Program I discussed in chapter 1 (Billings and Stoeckle 1977) simply collected responses from medical students who had gone through the GTA program.

16 The role that the NBME played in this is a fascinating and (as far as I'm aware) as-yet unanswered question. The NBME is a group of professional researchers in medical education, funded by the testing fees of the USMLE. These are quite high (see chapter 6).

17 "Although the conference focused on graduate medical education, the organizers and attendees recognized that the concepts, principles, and vocabulary apply across all levels of professional development, from undergraduate through continuing medical education" (Duffy et al. 2004:496–497).

18 Unit members tend to collectively publish on average of ten articles per year (about three per faculty member) and give around fourteen presentations at conferences. Unit members are collectively either principle investigator or co-PI on about five grants per year.

19 This kind of academic work is frequently more lucrative for social science and humanities doctorate-level scholars than positions in their own disciplinary departments might be. An assistant professor in such a unit could expect to earn, on average, about $98,000 per year in 2013, with an associate professor at $118,000 and a full professor at $148,000.

20 It is also telling for the positionality of GTA program vis-à-vis medical education research that every program I studied was either housed physically and organizationally within the hierarchy of a dedicated department *or* supervised by a physician affiliated with one.

21 I am struck by the statistics on race and pain management for children (Goyal et al. 2015) and those on race and maternal mortality (Creanga et al. 2015). These are people who, all other things being equal, will suffer and die because their Black bodies produce a reaction in a physician, *even with that physician's best efforts to control bias.* Likewise, I am struck by research in medical education on how marginalized medical trainees can and should respond to racism and sexism from their patients. I have been involved in medical education research on training medical students about transgender patients (Underman et al. 2016), and the evidence on "trans broken arm syndrome" is overwhelming.

CHAPTER 3. "THIS POWER WITH MY BODY"

1 I draw this term from Michelle Murphy's (2004) work on feminist self-help clinics and the pelvic self-examination. Playing on Donna Haraway's formulation of the modest witness as that gentleman scholar whose unimpeachable character serves

as his credible claim to objectivity, Murphy outlines the forms of knowledge production that occur when one's body becomes the object of study. She traces circuits of affect, materiality, and subject-making alongside scientific histories of objectivity.

2 Haptic sensory experiences are forms of touching and feeling that go beyond skin-deep to experiences of the body's interiority, awareness of its position in space, and feelings of pressure and motion (Paterson 2007).

3 Like other forms of intimate labor, GTA work is associated with forms of unpaid work that has historically been done by women. I make this claim on two fronts. First, the kinds of emotional skills that GTAs teach medical students have long been associated with women (good listening, caring, supporting emotions), and as such, it should be no surprise that women tend to do better on these skills in standardized tests (Cuddy et al. 2011). Second, as I laid out in the previous chapter, the work that GTAs do was once extracted by force or coercion from women on the assumption that it was owed to the medical profession, either by virtue of the social compact of the teaching hospital or in the name of scientific progress or public health. And, in fact, this work is still being extracted through the practice of pelvic exams on anesthetized patients (Friesen 2018).

4 While most sociologists will be familiar with work on emotional labor, "affective labor" provides a larger conceptual tent because it extends beyond the management of emotion to the production of affects and affective states in and of themselves (Hardt 1999; Hardt and Negri 2001; Mankekar and Gupta 2016; Vora 2010; Weeks 2007, 2011). Thus, affective labor captures the dimensions of paid work that require workers to manage their own and their clients' emotions, but it goes much further in that affective labor produces connections and new forms of sociality. As Michael Hardt argues, affective labor produces "social networks, forms of community, biopower. . . . In the production and reproduction of affects . . . collective subjectivities are produced and sociality is produced—even if those subjectivities and that sociality are directly exploitable by capital" (Hardt 1999:96–97).

5 When I was working as a GTA, I was able to effectively transfer from a program in one state to a program in another when I started graduate school. The techniques and the "script" stayed mostly the same. The biggest difference was learning to work with a partner.

6 GTAs call it the "script." Marie was the first GTA to name it as such to me. When I asked her what she meant, she explained, "The verbal component of the teaching . . . how you explain your curriculum. . . . There may be a set curriculum, but the way the different GTAs approach teaching the curriculum varies. . . . The script is not the same for every person, but it's a format and, you know, a skeleton that one person may use with . . . different teaching examples and different . . . explanations."

7 This happened to me once. I had been on the table in the morning for both sessions, expecting to be in the teaching role that afternoon. However, a GTA who had been scheduled to work was unable to make it due to a family emergency.

I agreed to stay on the table and teach solo in exchange for double pay. You can see the conundrum, then, for GTAs and directors. It was a lot of money (around $660, which was about a month's rent and utilities for me at the time), but also a lot of physical wear on the body and mental fatigue of having to be incredibly vigilant *while also* teaching.

8 I am aware of the deeply ironic and particularly the US-specific dynamic whereby people who make their livings as "professional patients" may be unable to access healthcare themselves due to its being unaffordable.

9 Medical school simulation centers often have cameras in the rooms in order to allow instructors or faculty to observe sessions, although cameras are never used during GTA sessions.

10 I suspect that this estimate, for the average GTA in Chicago, is probably low. Beth was working in a program that intentionally limited the number of times a GTA could have an exam per week to four. That means that she could have up to two hundred pelvic exams in a year. In Chicago, there are no such limitations. During a busy semester, a GTA might have as many as twelve pelvic exams in a single day. I have no reason to believe that the quality or depth of bodily knowledge in one would be more developed than in that other. I only want to note that GTAs' bodily knowledge is based on a *much* higher frequency of examination than an average person's would be (who might get one a year, if that).

11 GTAs all seem to work with the specter of the sexually motivated GTA in their narrative toolbox. I suspect that, given how hard early GTAs had to work to legitimize their work as explicitly not sex work (and thus avoid the same stigma and marginalization that sex workers experience), this narrative serves as an important form of boundary work for the profession. Beth said, "Sex work is a stigmatized kind of work in our society and patient instructors spend a lot of time trying to convince people not to stigmatize them in that way. . . . There's this strong motivation for trying to draw as bright a line as possible between the two." This kind of boundary work, however, seems purely outward-facing. Alex, for example, told me that a friend of his compared his being a GTA to prostitution. He was extremely upset by this remark and what it meant for both GTAs *and* sex workers: "Anyone who works with their body . . . that's somehow shameful. . . . Especially in our work, but in sex work as well . . . just the idea that if you're a prostitute, you're maybe some sort of desperate victim, and I guess we must be, too. . . . It's just like a completely off-base comment, in terms of sex work and also what we're doing." He further argued: "It's really not addressing the sort of political aspects that can be involved." Thus, while there is a strong motivation to construct a narrative of GTAs as a profession *contra* the work of sex work, some GTAs see parallels between the two as forms of work, in terms of stigma and exclusion. In fact, I spoke to at least two GTAs who were also working in various forms of sex work at the time.

12 This raises interesting questions about gender and sex assigned at birth as they operate within normative medical discourse. Programs that I am aware of that

include trans, nonbinary, and gender nonconforming GTAs bill themselves as such. The pelvic exam seems to remain very much normatively gendered, as women's healthcare in medical education. Any inclusion of gender beyond the binaristic assumptions of cisnormativity is marginalized as "special" or advanced training.

13 I mentioned in chapter 1 that most GTA programs disallow GTAs from teaching while menstruating. Some programs are stricter about this in order to avoid causing the medical students emotional distress. This is of course about taboos around menstruation, but it's also practical: some students can take the sight of blood as evidence that they have injured the GTA. This would then require *more* labor on the GTAs' part to reassure the students that everything is fine and normal.

14 The literature on this is too vast to adequately do justice to here, but I am in particular drawing on the work of Grosz (1994), Butler (2002), Fausto-Sterling (2000), Martin (2001), and others. Medicine has been intimately complicit in these constructions. In Michel Foucault's famous account in *The History of Sexuality*, once medicine could establish in the female body a "pathology intrinsic to it," it could be "integrated into the sphere of medical practices" (Foucault 1994:104).

15 "Signs increase in affective value as an effect of the movement between signs: the more signs circulate, the more affective they become" (Ahmed 2015:45).

16 Ahmed gives the example of Charles Darwin's response of disgust to the "naked savage," where both nakedness and lower social status become stuck to the body of the native. "Lowness" becomes an affectively charged sign.

17 See Giuffre and Williams (2000) about strategies for desexualizing intimate exams.

18 There is a growing body of work on the damaging effects of anti-fat bias among physicians (Foster et al. 2003; Jay et al. 2009; Sabin, Marini, and Nosek 2012; Schwartz et al. 2003; Teachman and Brownell 2001).

19 Of the forms of bodily labor identified by sociologists, only a few involve the worker's body as the site of paid labor. These include types of "display work" (Mears 2014), such as fashion modeling; various forms of sex work (Bernstein 2007; Hoang 2015; Mears 2014); egg and sperm donation (Almeling 2011), and surrogacy (Lewis 2016; Pande 2010). What these types of work share in common is some kind of traffic in affect: producing desire, circulating care. These also involve close attention to and selective detachment from the body. For example, surrogacy involves detailed cultivation of the worker's body and emotions to produce a healthy fetus—the surrogate must care for the fetus without becoming too emotionally bonded (Holzberg 2018; Pande 2010).

20 In a 2011 article in *Gender & Society* based on pilot data from this project, I outlined the strategies that GTAs use as intimate laborers to maintain authority and control in the teaching session. I argued that GTAs deploy what I term a "strategic dualism," which I defined as using constructions of the body as an object while simultaneously relying on subjective experiences.

21 The teres muscle is along the posterior wall of the axillary (armpit) region, which is palpated as part of the breast examination.

22　I struggled to find data to provide an estimate of how much this industry generates per year. Swanson and Roberts (2016) estimated that the entire USMLE generated $120 million in 2014. Using similar methodology—the fee posted on the USMLE website of $1,295 times reported MD and DO test-takers (United States Medical Licensing Examination n.d.)—I estimated that step 2 CS generated $45 million in fees in 2018.

23　The second study was a cost-effectiveness analysis done in 2013–2014 in the United Kingdom. I adjusted the cost to USD by using November 2014 rates for GBP.

24　Two things of note here. First, this study was done 1991–1993. In 2019 dollars this would be about $78,000. Second, simulated patients themselves were paid only $12,000. The rest went to faculty and administration.

CHAPTER 4. PRACTICING PROFESSIONALISM, PERFORMING AUTHENTICITY

1　For the curious, in medical simulation, the correct term is "manikin." A mannequin is what is used in clothing stores to model outfits. The difference between these words has to do with their language origins (Dutch versus French). Now you have a fun fact for your next dinner party.

2　There have been a few studies and pilot projects that explicitly attempt to use simulation to foster empathy in trainees (Batt-Rawden et al. 2013; Pedersen 2010; Wear and Varley 2008), but few studies consider the *routine* role of emotion in simulation.

3　The focus of this chapter will be on the ways in which simulation manages, harnesses, and produces emotion. For more on the measurement of emotion through simulation, see Teherani, Hauer, and O'Sullivan (2008).

4　The centrality of cadavers for emotional socialization has been challenged by scholars who have revisited these classic sites of professional training. Alexandra Vinson (2019) argues convincingly that the central task of professional socialization in today's cadaver lab is allowing medical students to "play" with the identity of being a surgeon and to learn how to interact with peers.

5　This emphasis on professionalism in medical training as a "third pillar" is a recent development, and professionalism must be understood as a culturally contingent set of practices. Professionalism, therefore, is an account the medical profession has developed of itself to justify continued professional dominance.

6　Handwashing is on the checklist that GTAs use to indicate whether the student passed the encounter, and it is one of the things many simulated patient encounters grade them on as well.

7　This contrast is curious and may be related to comfort with sexuality, but it may also be related to methodology. I identified myself as a GTA to the GTAs I interviewed, thus making me an insider. I did not do this for medical students. Indeed, medical students at the schools I studied are very often subject to surveys, interviews, and focus groups by medical education researchers at their university.

There may have been some nervousness about my role as a researcher. There is also simply quite a lot of anxiety for medical students about how they are being evaluated by superiors and outsiders.

8 In a fascinating study, researchers examined the impact of simulation of the breast exam on students' ability to locate pathology, with a particular interest in the role of shame (Hautz et al. 2017). One group of students examined rubber models and the other group examined the real breast of a simulated patient. Both groups then examined a rubber model worn by a simulated patient that simulated several types of pathologies (i.e., lumps and bumps). The researchers measured students' levels of shame before the intervention (i.e., examining the rubber model or the real person) and then again at the assessment. The group that had not practiced on a real person had increased levels of shame. They also spent less time with the simulated patient in the assessment and located fewer of the simulated abnormalities. The researchers concluded that working on a real person caused students to have to *work through* their feelings of shame about the exam. While this didn't lead to a statistically significant decline in shame, it did allow them to spend more time in the assessment and locate more pathologies. In short, students who work through their feelings do a better job on intimate exams.

9 Terri Kapsalis and others (including myself and some of the GTAs I interviewed) have compared the work that GTAs do to the work that sex workers do. In both contexts, we have a someone—in this case, a cisgender woman—allowing a stranger access to her body while she performs labor to regulate her and that stranger's experience of the encounter. While sex work is inherently sexual but the work GTAs do is intentionally desexualized, the affective labor of balancing between authenticity and artificiality is theoretically similar to what sociologist Elizabeth Bernstein has called "bounded authenticity" (2007), by which she means a genuine emotional and physical encounter that is almost bounded in time and emotional depth.

10 For a discussion of this, see Teherani et al. (2008), Wear and Varley (2008), Berg et al. (2011a, 2011b), and Underman and Hirshfield (2016).

11 I suspect, in part, this may speak to the limitations of snowball sampling and self-selected participation. Students who had a positive experience with the GTA session and who were reflexive about it were probably more likely to speak with me.

CHAPTER 5. "WHAT DOES IT MEAN TO RELAX YOUR HAND?"

1 The specificity of context for sensation is important to note in this example. Recall Marie discussing guiding sexual partners around and to her cervix in chapter 3. The sensations conjured by touching a cervix with one's hands during sex may be similar to those of doing a bimanual exam, but for the expert, these two ways of feeling must be disentangled.

2 Medical sociologists and those working in fields close to ours are more than comfortable describing the patient's body as an object constructed under the medical gaze. Foucault (1994) shows how the reorganization of knowledge, practice, and

space allowed for our contemporary episteme of medical knowledge to come into being during the seventeenth through nineteenth centuries. Practices such as bringing patients into the hospital and dissecting corpses allowed physicians to locate disease in the body and, as this episteme more fully developed, in particular parts of the body. As a result, the patient's subjectivity gradually receded into the background as diagnostic and therapeutic technologies expanded during the twentieth century. There is therefore a dichotomy between "an objective, public and scientific way of knowing the body from the outside" and a "subjective, private and personal way of knowing the body from the inside" (Mol and Law 2004:44–45). Physicians are thoroughly trained in the first mode of knowing and have no truck with the second. Or so the story goes. More recently, though, scholars have begun to attend to the ways in which the physician's body is also socially constructed. These sets of literature engage with the physician's body and its senses to understand how medical trainees rely upon their own bodily feelings to do the work of the clinical encounter (Hammer 2018; Harris 2016). The legacy of Foucault's medical gaze has often meant that the sense of sight and medical ways of seeing are privileged in such literatures, but scholars are also examining how senses of hearing, taste, smell, and, most importantly, touch, are honed through medical training. In this formulation, as medical trainees move from trainees to expert, their bodies undergo an open-ended process in which their dispositions and modes of perceiving the world—and the instruments and other bodies present in the clinic—are shaped for medical work. The trainee must become aware of and learn to draw on bodily sensations in ways specific to the work of clinical medicine (Harris 2016). The body, thus, is enacted in practice (Mol and Law 2004).

3 Much of the theorizing on this topic relies upon the *Phenomenology of Perception* and related works by philosopher Maurice Merleau-Ponty (2013). Merleau-Ponty was concerned with the tradition in philosophy dating back to Rene Descartes (of "I think therefor I am" fame) to split us all into thinking, knowing, rational minds and bodies as objects or vehicles for driving our thinking, knowing minds around all day. Merleau-Ponty sought to decenter language as the primary locus of cognition and instead locate our foundational relationality to the world around us in our bodies ("being-in-the-world"). Merleau-Ponty uses the corporeal or body schema to describe a unified sensory locus through which embodied experience of the world produces cognition.

4 Massumi (2002) calls these two sides the "virtual" and the "real."

5 These are looking, touching, tapping, and listening, respectively.

6 See Butler (2011) on materialization. What Barad adds to this is the idea that matter acts back on discourse. While the idea that objects have agency is at this point quite a comfortable claim for science and technology studies, I suspect it will be a more controversial claim for sociologists.

7 Barad draws from the philosopher-physicist Niels Bohr. Bohr proposed a type of experiment that would demonstrate that how you measure light's behavior

will shape what you actually find. In classic Newtonian physics, the interference of measurement (such as a radar gun) can be calculated and made negligible. In Bohr's work, the conditions of measurement are part of the object. She uses Bohr's thought experiment about measuring the momentum and position of an electron. To measure momentum, you need a platform that moves to gauge the motion. To measure position, you need a platform that does not move to gauge where impact happens. You cannot measure both simultaneously. This means that objects do not preexist with determinable properties just waiting for the right measurement tool, but that measurement actually determines the outcome. A slightly less complicated and probably more familiar example is Schrodinger's poor cat. In this thought experiment, a cat is placed in a totally sound-proof box and a gun is programmed to either fire or not fire at random. The cat is both dead and alive until the experimenter opens the box and checks (i.e., measures the cat's outcome). Now go hug your pets.

8 See Prentice (2013) on objectification.

9 I am thinking of the pelvic exam as an "apparatus" in the sense that Barad (2007) uses the term from Foucault. For Barad, an apparatus is a given configuration of materiality and discourse that sets the conditions of possibility for subjects and objects. Apparatuses are "boundary-drawing practices" (Barad 2007:140) that enact what configurations of materiality matter and which do not.

10 GTAs might focus their attention on an ovary during mittelschmerz (which is a really fun word to say but not a fun thing to experience) or the mid-cycle pain associated with ovulation. While in this configuration the ovary becomes an object, it is not the same kind of object. It is not a pedagogical tool for training medical students in the pelvic exam. The twinge or pain associated is not a register of correct or incorrect technique.

11 Speculum size is important because vaginal walls have differing amounts of elasticity. A person who has given birth vaginally, for example, might need a wider bill to fully support their vaginal walls. Part of GTAs' knowing their own bodies is knowing what size speculum makes it easiest for students to see their cervices. As I said in chapter 3, medical schools usually provide the materials to GTAs. Medical schools have the same issues as any other organization and sometimes through human error, the speculum size a GTA prefers isn't available. This means that GTAs must adapt their teaching in the moment to what's available. They often use this to teach medical students how to adjust their speculum insertion technique in case the specula available aren't ideal.

12 There is an interesting question here about just how nonstandard the body of a GTA can be. Recall in chapter 3 that Gretchen felt proud of using her queer, fat body to teach medical students. Fatness is often introduced in the GTA session as another bodily variation that requires physicians to adjust their technique. Other kinds of variation, such as in gender presentation, seem less welcome. Outside of training contexts specific to transgender health, I have not heard any explicit mention in GTA sessions of that fact that men might have a uterus, for example.

Anatomical diversity, it seems, is considered an educational advantage, while perhaps social, cultural, or political variation might not be in this context. That said, I do not have the data to back up this claim. Likewise, there are no national studies that I am aware of that assess diversity by race, gender, sexuality, disability, or religion among simulated patients.

13 I found no patterns in my data about gender or the sex assigned to the medical student at birth in relationship to nervousness or confidence with the pelvic exam. Some medical students who had had pelvic exams before were more nervous, others were less. Those without this kind of anatomy were equally nervous or not nervous, depending on their lack of previous experience. Likewise, GTAs expressed opinions equally on both sides as to who performed better. Some GTAs thought those who'd had pelvic exams before would do worse because they might think the exam is supposed to hurt, while other GTAs thought they'd do better because they understand the vulnerability of the experience. This lack of finding is curious, but I suspect that it has to do with the *clinical* component of the pelvic exam: having to perform with competence a task that is medicalized.

14 For example, Jasbir Puar (2007) writes of the body-as-assemblage via understanding the turban-wearing Sikh. The Sikh's body is comprised of different components, including the signature turban, which bind him to other bodies, social arrangements, and emotions. The turban is read as a symbol of terrorism via American history and culture, and thus the turban assembles the body of the Sikh as a figure of terror.

15 This process is often called "articulation" in the science and technology studies literature (Harris 2016; Latour 2004; Prentice 2013).

16 See Nick Crossley's article linking the concepts of habit and habitus: "Habit involves a modification and enlargement of the corporeal schema, an incorporation of new 'principles' of action and know-how that permit new ways of acting and understanding. . . . It is a sediment of past activity that remains alive in the present in the form of the structures of the corporeal schema; shaping perception, conception, deliberation, emotion, and action" (2001:104).

17 See Monica Casper's work on fetal surgery (1998).

CHAPTER 6. NOT JUST BONES, ORGANS, AND SCIENCE

1 Narrative medicine comes from the academic field of literature and uses storytelling and literary analysis to foster empathy and understanding (Charon 2001, 2008). It was popularized by Rita Charon, who holds both an MD and a PhD in English.

2 In addition to my work on GTA programs, I had the opportunity to observe several years' worth of "advanced patient scenarios" during my postdoctoral work. These scenarios are day-long workshops for third- or fourth-year medical students allowing them to encounter simulated patients who are roleplaying various types of challenges to the physician-patient relationship. These encounters occur in a classroom and are group-based so that students can share techniques

and tips with each other and discuss such methods of providing care with their faculty. Examples of encounters are domestic violence, vaccine refusal, or angry patients. See Underman et al. (2016) for an example of a case I worked on that involved transgender patients. Observing these workshops really allowed me to see how trainees wrestle with the need to assert medical authority while maintaining a patient-centered approach.

3 There is quite a lot of literature comparing and contrasting Foucault's work on technologies of the self with Bourdieu's work on the habitus (Burkitt 2002; Decoteau 2013; McNay 1999). I do not mean to lightly mix sets of theorists here. Rather, I agree that these concepts have much in common and also that there are important distinctions. I use the term "technologies" here because it more suitably connects microlevel practices to knowledge and power. I incorporate work on capital to describe the sets of attributes that are cultivated by these technologies. I have no interest here in theorizing a habitus of patient empowerment, but that work could be done elsewhere. Affect and the habitus have likewise been adeptly connected by other scholars (Blackman 2013; Gould 2009).

4 Unfortunately, the practice of examining anesthetized patients without their consent isn't as much of a relic of the past as Sergei frames it. See the conclusion to this book.

5 In her work on "mothercraft" and how birth-workers foster empowered birthing for some patients and not others, sociologist Katharine McCabe argues: "This mode of empowerment is delimited by women's individual purchasing power making it distinct from feminist health ideals of an earlier era in that it is individualistic, consumeristic, and a-political and exacerbates social divisions between women according to their consumer viability, lifestyle choices, and cultural health capital leaving those who do not or cannot 'choose' at the margins" (2016:183).

6 For a breakdown of what countries require testing of clinical skills, see Price et al. (2018).

CONCLUSION

1 This practice was also the subject of an article in the August 2019 issue of *Elle Magazine*.

2 A good example of this is the anguish and hope provoked by the introduction of devices such as tablets and computers into the clinic as electronic health records become standard. Medical educators see the promise of such technologies but must invent new ways to train medical students to divide their attention between the computer screen and the patient. Where do you look, for example, while taking a history? How do you position your body to appear attentive to the patient while also typing notes?

BIBLIOGRAPHY

AAMC—*See* Association of American Medical Colleges.

Abrahamson, Stephen. 1960. "The Professional Educator and Medical Education." *Journal of Higher Education* 31(1):38–41.

Adashi, Eli Y. 2019. "JAMA Forum: Teaching Pelvic Examination under Anesthesia without Patient Consent." *News@JAMA*. https://newsatjama.jama.com.

Ahmed, Sara. 2015. *The Cultural Politics of Emotion*. New York: Routledge.

Ahmed, Sara. 2004. "Affective Economies." *Social Text* 22(2):117–139.

Almeling, Rene. 2011. *Sex Cells: The Medical Market for Eggs and Sperm*. Berkeley: University of California Press.

Altbach, Philip G., and Robert Cohen. 1990. "American Student Activism: The Post-Sixties Transformation." *Journal of Higher Education* 61(1):32–49.

Anderson, Ben. 2012. "Affect and Biopower: Towards a Politics of Life." *Transactions of the Institute of British Geographers* 37(1):28–43.

Anderson, M. Brownell. 1993. "Proceedings of the AAMC's Consensus Conference on the Use of Standardized Patients in the Teaching and Evaluation of Clinical Skills." *Academic Medicine* 68(6):437–484.

Anderson, Robert M., Martha M. Funnell, Patricia M. Butler, Marilynn S. Arnold, James T. Fitzgerald, and Catherine C. Feste. 1995. "Patient Empowerment: Results of a Randomized Controlled Trial." *Diabetes Care* 18(7):943–949.

Annandale, Ellen. 2014. *The Sociology of Health and Medicine: A Critical Introduction*. Cambridge, UK: Polity Press.

Anon. n.d. "Sign the Petition." *End Step 2 CS*. http://endstep2cs.com (retrieved May 26, 2019).

Archer, Julian, Nick Lynn, Lee Coombes, Martin Roberts, Tom Gale, Tristan Price, and Sam Regan de Bere. 2016. "The Impact of Large-Scale Licensing Examinations in Highly Developed Countries: A Systematic Review." *BMC Medical Education* 16(1):212–222.

Armstrong, David. 1995. "The Rise of Surveillance Medicine." *Sociology of Health & Illness* 17(3):393–404.

Armstrong, David. 1983. *Political Anatomy of the Body: Medical Knowledge in Britain in the Twentieth Century*. Cambridge, UK: Cambridge University Press.

Association of American Medical Colleges. 2016. "The State of Women in Academic Medicine: The Pipeline and Pathways to Leadership, 2015–2016." https://www.aamc.org.

Association of Professors of Gynecology and Obstetrics. 2008. "The Pelvic Exam." *APGO Clinical Skills Curriculum*. Crofton, MD.

Bakker, Isabella. 2007. "Social Reproduction and the Constitution of a Gendered Political Economy." *New Political Economy* 12(4):541–556.

Balint, Enid. 1969. "The Possibilities of Patient-Centered Medicine." *Journal of the Royal College of General Practitioners* 17(82):269–276.

Balint, Michael. 1957. *The Doctor, His Patient and the Illness*. London: Churchill Livingstone.

Bannow, Tara. 2010. "Med School Changes Pelvic Exam Instruction." *Minnesota Daily*, February 17.

Barad, Karen. 2012. "On Touching—The Inhuman that Therefore I Am." *Differences* 23(3):206–223.

Barad, Karen. 2007. *Meeting the Universe Halfway: Quantum Physics and the Entanglement of Matter and Meaning*. Durham, NC: Duke University Press.

Barker-Benfield, Graham John. 2004. *The Horrors of the Half-Known Life: Male Attitudes toward Women and Sexuality in 19th-Century America*. New York: Routledge.

Barnes, Alan J., Walter G. Chappell, Richard E. Darnell, Michael Williams, and Hilliard Jason. 1970. "Controversy and Trends in Medical Education. Report of the 8th Annual Conference on Research on Medical Education." *Social Science & Medicine* 4(6):677–679.

Barrios, Roberto E. 2017. *Governing Affect: Neoliberalism and Disaster Reconstruction*. Lincoln: University of Nebraska Press.

Barrows, Howard S., and Stephen Abrahamson. 1964. "The Programmed Patient: A Technique for Appraising Student Performance in Clinical Neurology." *Academic Medicine* 39(8):802–805.

Barry, Michael J., and Susan Edgman-Levitan. 2012. "Shared Decision Making—The Pinnacle of Patient-Centered Care." *New England Journal of Medicine* 366(9):780–781.

Batt-Rawden, Samantha A., Margaret S. Chisolm, Blair Anton, and Tabor E. Flickinger. 2013. "Teaching Empathy to Medical Students: An Updated, Systematic Review." *Academic Medicine* 88(8):1171–1177.

Beach, Mary Catherine, Mary Rosner, Lisa A. Cooper, Patrick S. Duggan, and John Shatzer. 2007. "Can Patient-Centered Attitudes Reduce Racial and Ethnic Disparities in Care?" *Academic Medicine* 82(2):193–198.

Becker, Howard Saul. 2002. *Boys in White: Student Culture in Medical School*. Piscataway, NJ: Transaction Publishers.

Beckmann, C. R. B., G. H. Lipscomb, L. Williford, E. Bryant, and F. W. Ling. 1992. "Gynaecological Teaching Associates in the 1990s." *Medical Education* 26(2):105–109.

Beckmann, Charles R. B., B. M. Barzansky, B. F. Sharf, and K. Meyers. 1988. "Training Gynaecological Teaching Associates." *Medical Education* 22(2):124–131.

Beckmann, Charles R. B., William N. Spellacy, Annette Yonke, Barbara Barzansky, and Raima P. Cunningham. 1985. "Initial Instruction in the Pelvic Examination in the

United States and Canada, 1983." *American Journal of Obstetrics and Gynecology* 151(1):58–60.

Bell, Susan E. 2019. "Interpreter Assemblages: Caring for Immigrant and Refugee Patients in US Hospitals." *Social Science & Medicine* 226:29–36.

Bell, Susan E. 2009. *DES Daughters, Embodied Knowledge, and the Transformation of Women's Health Politics in the Late Twentieth Century.* Philadelphia: Temple University Press.

Bell, Susan. 1979. "Political Gynecology: Gynecological Imperialism and the Politics of Self-Help." *Science for the People* 11(5):8–14.

Bell, Susan E., and Anne E. Figert. 2012. "Medicalization and Pharmaceuticalization at the Intersections: Looking Backward, Sideways and Forward." *Social Science & Medicine* 75(5):775–783.

Bensing, Jozien. 2000. "Bridging the Gap: The Separate Worlds of Evidence-Based Medicine and Patient-Centered Medicine." *Patient Education and Counseling* 39(1):17–25.

Berg, Katherine, Benjamin Blatt, Joseph Lopreiato, Julianna Jung, Arielle Schaeffer, Daniel Heil, Tamara Owens, Pamela L. Carter-Nolan, Dale Berg, and Jon Veloski. 2015. "Standardized Patient Assessment of Medical Student Empathy: Ethnicity and Gender Effects in a Multi-Institutional Study." *Academic Medicine* 90(1):105–111.

Berg, Katherine, Joseph F. Majdan, Dale Berg, Jon Veloski, and Mohammadreza Hojat. 2011a. "A Comparison of Medical Students' Self-Reported Empathy with Simulated Patients' Assessments of the Students' Empathy." *Medical Teacher* 33(5):388–391.

Berg, Katherine, Joseph F. Majdan, Dale Berg, Jon Veloski, and Mohammadreza Hojat. 2011b. "Medical Students' Self-Reported Empathy and Simulated Patients' Assessments of Student Empathy: An Analysis by Gender and Ethnicity." *Academic Medicine* 86(8):984–988.

Berg, Marc. 1995. "Turning a Practice into a Science: Reconceptualizing Postwar Medical Practice." *Social Studies of Science* 25(3):437–476.

Bernstein, Elizabeth. 2007. *Temporarily Yours: Intimacy, Authenticity, and the Commerce of Sex.* Chicago: University of Chicago Press.

Billings, J. Andrew, and John D. Stoeckle. 1977. "Pelvic Examination Instruction and the Doctor-Patient Relationship." *Journal of Medical Education* 52(10):834–839.

Blackman, Lisa. 2013. "Habit and Affect: Revitalizing a Forgotten History." *Body & Society* 19(2–3):186–216.

Blanch-Hartigan, Danielle. 2012. "An Effective Training to Increase Accurate Recognition of Patient Emotion Cues." *Patient Education and Counseling* 89(2):274–280.

Blanch-Hartigan, Danielle, Susan A. Andrzejewski, and Krista M. Hill. 2012. "The Effectiveness of Training to Improve Person Perception Accuracy: A Meta-Analysis." *Basic and Applied Social Psychology* 34(6):483–498.

Blanch-Hartigan, Danielle, and Mollie A. Ruben. 2013. "Training Clinicians to Accurately Perceive Their Patients: Current State and Future Directions." *Patient Education and Counseling* 92(3):328–336.

Bloom, Samuel W. 1988. "Structure and Ideology in Medical Education: An Analysis of Resistance to Change." *Journal of Health and Social Behavior* 29(4): 294–306.

Bloomfield, Hanna E., Andrew Olson, Nancy Greer, Amy Cantor, Roderick Mac-Donald, Indulis Rutks, and Timothy J. Wilt. 2014. "Screening Pelvic Examinations in Asymptomatic, Average-Risk Adult Women: An Evidence Report for a Clinical Practice Guideline from the American College of Physicians." *Annals of Internal Medicine* 161(1):46–53.

Bonilla-Silva, Eduardo. 2019. "Feeling Race: Theorizing the Racial Economy of Emotions." *American Sociological Review* 84(1):1–25.

Boris, Eileen, and Rhacel Salazar Parreñas. 2010. *Intimate Labors: Cultures, Technologies, and the Politics of Care.* Palo Alto, CA: Stanford University Press.

Bosk, Charles L., Mary Dixon-Woods, Christine A. Goeschel, and Peter J. Pronovost. 2009. "Reality Check for Checklists." *The Lancet* 374(9688):P444–445.

Bourdieu, Pierre. 2000. *Pascalian Meditations.* Palo Alto, CA: Stanford University Press.

Bourdieu, Pierre. 1977. *Outline of a Theory of Practice.* Cambridge, UK: Cambridge University Press.

Bourgois, Philippe, Seth M. Holmes, Kim Sue, and James Quesada. 2017. "Structural Vulnerability: Operationalizing the Concept to Address Health Disparities in Clinical Care." *Academic Medicine: Journal of the Association of American Medical Colleges* 92(3):299–307.

Braveman, Paula A., Shiriki Kumanyika, Jonathan Fielding, Thomas LaVeist, Luisa N. Borrell, Ron Manderscheid, and Adewale Troutman. 2011. "Health Disparities and Health Equity: The Issue Is Justice." *American Journal of Public Health* 101(S1):S149–S155.

Briggs, Laura. 2003. *Reproducing Empire.* Berkeley, CA: University of California Press.

Brosnan, Caragh. 2010. "Making Sense of Differences between Medical Schools through Bourdieu's Concept of 'Field.'" *Medical Education* 44(7):645–652.

Brosnan, Caragh. 2009. "Pierre Bourdieu and the Theory of Medical Education: Thinking 'Relationally' about Medical Students and Medical Curricula." Pp. 65–82 in *Handbook of the Sociology of Medical Education*, edited by Caragh Brosnan and Bryan S. Turner. London: Routledge.

Brown, Nik. 2015. "Metrics of Hope: Disciplining Affect in Oncology." *Health* 19(2):119–136.

Buchbinder, Mara, and Stefan Timmermans. 2014. "Affective Economies and the Politics of Saving Babies' Lives." *Public Culture* 26(1):101–126.

Buck, George H. 1991. "Development of Simulators in Medical Education." *Gesnerus* 48:7–28.

Burkitt, Ian. 2002. "Technologies of the Self: Habitus and Capacities." *Journal for the Theory of Social Behaviour* 32(2):219–237.

Bury, Michael. 1982. "Chronic Illness as Biographical Disruption." *Sociology of Health & Illness* 4(2):167–182.

Buse, Christina, Daryl Martin, and Sarah Nettleton. 2018. "Conceptualising 'Materialities of Care': Making Visible Mundane Material Culture in Health and Social Care Contexts." *Sociology of Health & Illness* 40(2):243–255.

Butler, Judith. 2011. *Bodies that Matter: On the Discursive Limits of Sex*. New York: Routledge.

Butler, Judith. 2002. *Gender Trouble*. New York: Routledge.

Cantillon, Peter, Brian Stewart, Karolien Haeck, James Bills, Jean Ker, and Jan-Joost Rethans. 2010. "Simulated Patient Programmes in Europe: Collegiality or Separate Development?" *Medical Teacher* 32(3):e106–110.

Casper, Monica J. 1998. *The Making of the Unborn Patient*. New Brunswick, NJ: Rutgers University Press.

Casper, Monica J., and Adele E. Clarke. 1998. "Making the Pap Smear into 'The Right Tool' for the Job: Cervical Cancer Screening in the USA, circa 1940–95." *Social Studies of Science* 28(2):255–290.

Charles, Cathy, Amiram Gafni, and Tim Whelan. 1997. "Shared Decision-Making in the Medical Encounter: What Does It Mean? (Or It Takes at Least Two to Tango)." *Social Science & Medicine* 44(5):681–692.

Charon, Rita. 2008. *Narrative Medicine: Honoring the Stories of Illness*. New York: Oxford University Press.

Charon, Rita. 2001. "Narrative Medicine: Form, Function, and Ethics." *Annals of Internal Medicine* 134(1):83–87.

Clarke, Adele. 2005. *Situational Analysis: Grounded Theory after the Postmodern Turn*. New York: Sage.

Clarke, Adele E., and Joan H. Fujimura. 2014. *The Right Tools for the Job: At Work in Twentieth-Century Life Sciences*. Princeton, NJ: Princeton University Press.

Clarke, Adele E., Janet K. Shim, Laura Mamo, Jennifer Ruth Fosket, and Jennifer R. Fishman. 2003. "Biomedicalization: Technoscientific Transformations of Health, Illness, and U.S. Biomedicine." *American Sociological Review* 68(2):161–194.

Clough, Patricia T. 2008. "The Affective Turn: Political Economy, Biomedia and Bodies." *Theory, Culture & Society* 25(1):1–22.

Clough, Patricia Ticineto. 2003. "Affect and Control: Rethinking the Body 'beyond Sex and Gender.'" *Feminist Theory* 4(3):359–364.

Clough, Patricia Ticineto, Greg Goldberg, Rachel Schiff, Aaron Weeks, and Craig Willse. 2007. "Notes towards a Theory of Affect-Itself." *Ephemera: Theory and Politics in Organization* 7(1):60–77.

Clough, Patricia Ticineto, and Jean Halley, eds. 2007. *The Affective Turn: Theorizing the Social*. Durham, NC: Duke University Press Books.

Cohen, Devra S., Jerry A. Colliver, Michelle S. Marcy, Ethan D. Fried, and Mark H. Swartz. 1996. "Psychometric Properties of a Standardized-Patient Checklist and Rating-Scale Form Used to Assess Interpersonal and Communication Skills." *Academic Medicine: Journal of the Association of American Medical Colleges* 71(1 Suppl):S87–89.

Collins, Harry, and Robert Evans. 2008. *Rethinking Expertise*. Chicago: University of Chicago Press.

Cook, Catherine, and Margaret Brunton. 2015. "Pastoral Power and Gynaecological Examinations: A Foucauldian Critique of Clinician Accounts of Patient-Centred Consent." *Sociology of Health & Illness* 37(4):545–560.

Coole, Diana, and Samantha Frost. 2010. *New Materialisms: Ontology, Agency, and Politics*. Durham, NC: Duke University Press.

Cooper, Melinda, and Catherine Waldby. 2014. *Clinical Labor: Tissue Donors and Research Subjects in the Global Bioeconomy*. Durham, NC: Duke University Press.

Cox, Nicole, and Silvia Federici. 1976. *Counter-Planning from the Kitchen: Wages for Housework, a Perspective on Capital and the Left*. New York Wages for Housework Committee.

Craciun, Mariana. 2018. "Emotions and Knowledge in Expert Work: A Comparison of Two Psychotherapies." *American Journal of Sociology* 123(4):959–1003.

Crawford, Cecelia L., Anna Omery, and Jean Ann Seago. 2012. "The Challenges of Nurse-Physician Communication: A Review of the Evidence." *Journal of Nursing Administration* 42(12):548–550.

Creanga, Andreea A., Cynthia J. Berg, Carla Syverson, Kristi Seed, F. Carol Bruce, and William M. Callaghan. 2015. "Pregnancy-Related Mortality in the United States, 2006–2010." *Obstetrics & Gynecology* 125(1):5–12.

Crossley, Michele L., and Nick Crossley. 2001. "Patient Voices, Social Movements and the Habitus: How Psychiatric Survivors Speak Out." *Social Science & Medicine* 52(10):1477–1489.

Crossley, Nick. 2001. "The Phenomenological Habitus and Its Construction." *Theory and Society* 30(1):81–120.

Cuddy, Monica M., Kimberly A. Swygert, David B. Swanson, and Ann C. Jobe. 2011. "A Multilevel Analysis of Examinee Gender, Standardized Patient Gender, and United States Medical Licensing Examination Step 2 Clinical Skills Communication and Interpersonal Skills Scores." *Academic Medicine* 86(10):S17–S20.

Curran, Mallory, Edward Paul, and Liz Tobin Tyler. 2017. "The Medical-Legal Partnership Approach to Teaching Social Determinants of Health and Structural Competency in Residency Programs." *Academic Medicine* 92(3):292–298.

Daston, Lorraine. 1995. "The Moral Economy of Science." *Osiris* 10:2–24.

Davis, Kathy. 2007. *The Making of Our Bodies, Ourselves: How Feminism Travels across Borders*. Durham, NC: Duke University Press.

Davis, Margery H., Indika Karunathilake, and Ronald M. Harden. 2005. "AMEE Education Guide No. 28: The Development and Role of Departments of Medical Education." *Medical Teacher* 27(8):665–675.

Decoteau, Claire Laurier. 2013. *Ancestors and Antiretrovirals: The Biopolitics of HIV/AIDS in Post-Apartheid South Africa*. Chicago: University of Chicago Press.

de la Bellacasa, Maria Puig. 2011. "Matters of Care in Technoscience: Assembling Neglected Things." *Social Studies of Science* 41(1):85–106.

DeLanda, Manuel. 2019. *A New Philosophy of Society: Assemblage Theory and Social Complexity*. New York: Bloomsbury.

Deleuze, Gilles. 1992. "Postscript on the Societies of Control." *October* 59:3–7.

Deleuze, Gilles, and Félix Guattari. 1987. *A Thousand Plateaus: Capitalism and Schizophrenia*. Translated by Brian Massumi. Minneapolis: University of Minnesota Press.

Devellennes, Charles, and Benoît Dillet. 2018. "Questioning New Materialisms: An Introduction." *Theory, Culture & Society* 35(7–8):5–20.

DiMatteo, M. Robin, Ron D. Hays, and Louise M. Prince. 1986. "Relationship of Physicians' Nonverbal Communication Skill to Patient Satisfaction, Appointment Noncompliance, and Physician Workload." *Health Psychology* 5(6):581–594.

DiMatteo, M. Robin, Angelo Taranta, Howard S. Friedman, and Louise M. Prince. 1980. "Predicting Patient Satisfaction from Physicians' Nonverbal Communication Skills." *Medical Care* 18(4)376–387.

Ducey, Ariel. 2010. "Technologies of Caring Labor." Pp. 18–32 in *Intimate Labors: Cultures, Technologies, and the Politics of Care*, edited by Eileen Boris and Rhacel Salazar Parreñas. Palo Alto, CA: Stanford University Press.

Duffy, F. Daniel, Geoffrey H. Gordon, Gerald Whelan, Kathy Cole-Kelly, and Richard Frankel. 2004. "Assessing Competence in Communication and Interpersonal Skills: The Kalamazoo II Report." *Academic Medicine* 79(6):495–507.

Dugoff, Lorraine, Archana Pradhan, Petra Casey, John L. Dalrymple, Jodi F. Abbott, Samantha D. Buery-Joyner, Alice Chuang, Amie J. Cullimore, David A. Forstein, and Brittany S. Hampton. 2016. "Pelvic and Breast Examination Skills Curricula in United States Medical Schools: A Survey of Obstetrics and Gynecology Clerkship Directors." *BMC Medical Education* 16(1):314–320.

Ebeling, Mary F. E. 2016. *Healthcare and Big Data*. New York: Springer.

Ebert, Robert H. 1986. "Medical Education at the Peak of the Era of Experimental Medicine." *Daedalus* 115(2):55–81.

Edmiston, E. Kale. 2018. "Community-Led Peer Advocacy for Transgender Healthcare Access in the Southeastern United States: The Trans Buddy Program." Pp. 185–201 in *Healthcare in Motion: Immobilities in Health Service Delivery and Access*, edited by Cecilia Vindrola-Padros, Ginger A. Johnson, and Anne. E. Pfister. New York: Berghahn.

Elwyn, Glyn, Dominick Frosch, Richard Thomson, Natalie Joseph-Williams, Amy Lloyd, Paul Kinnersley, Emma Cording, Dave Tomson, Carole Dodd, and Stephen Rollnick. 2012. "Shared Decision Making: A Model for Clinical Practice." *Journal of General Internal Medicine* 27(10):1361–1367.

Emerson, Joan. 1970. "Behavior in Private Places: Sustaining Definitions of Reality in Gynecological Examinations." Pp. 247–260 in *The Production of Reality: Essays and Readings on Social Interaction*, edited by Jodi O'Brien. Los Angeles, CA: SAGE.

Epstein, Jennifer. 2010. "An Intimate Exam." *Inside Higher Ed*, February 19.

Epstein, Ronald M. 2007. "Assessment in Medical Education." *New England Journal of Medicine* 356(4):387–396.

Epstein, Steven. 2008. "Patient Groups and Health Movements." Pp. 499–539 in *The Handbook of Science and Technology Studies*, vol. 3, edited by Edward J. Hackett, Olga Amsterdamska, Michael Lynch, and Judy Wacjam. Cambridge, MA: MIT Press.

Evans, Robert. 2008. "The Sociology of Expertise: The Distribution of Social Fluency." *Sociology Compass* 2(1):281–298.

Eyal, Gil. 2013. "For a Sociology of Expertise: The Social Origins of the Autism Epidemic." *American Journal of Sociology* 118(4):863–907.

Fang, Wei Li, Paula J. Hillard, Richard W. Lindsay, and Paul B. Underwood. 1984. "Evaluation of Students' Clinical and Communication Skills in Performing a Gynecologic Examination." *Journal of Medical Education* 59(9):758–760.

Fausto-Sterling, Anne. 2000. *Sexing the Body: Gender Politics and the Construction of Sexuality*. New York: Basic Books.

Federation of State Medical Boards of the United States and National Board of Medical Examiners. 2019. "Step 2 Clinical Skills (CS): Content Description and General Information." https://www.usmle.org.

Fee, Elizabeth. 1975. "Women and Health Care: A Comparison of Theories." *International Journal of Health Services* 5(3):397–415.

Fenton, Joshua J., Anthony F. Jerant, Klea D. Bertakis, and Peter Franks. 2012. "The Cost of Satisfaction: A National Study of Patient Satisfaction, Health Care Utilization, Expenditures, and Mortality." *Archives of Internal Medicine* 172(5):405–411.

Finnerty, Edward P., Sheila Chauvin, Giulia Bonaminio, Mark Andrews, Robert G. Carroll, and Louis N. Pangaro. 2010. "Flexner Revisited: The Role and Value of the Basic Sciences in Medical Education." *Academic Medicine* 85(2):349–355.

Foster, Gary D., Thomas A. Wadden, Angela P. Makris, Duncan Davidson, Rebecca Swain Sanderson, David B. Allison, and Amy Kessler. 2003. "Primary Care Physicians' Attitudes about Obesity and Its Treatment." *Obesity Research* 11(10):1168–1177.

Foucault, Michel. 1995. *Discipline & Punish: The Birth of the Prison*. New York: Vintage Books.

Foucault, Michel. 1994. *The Birth of the Clinic: An Archaeology of Medical Perception*. New York: Vintage.

Foucault, Michel. 1990. *The History of Sexuality, Vol. 1: An Introduction*. Reissue edition. New York: Vintage.

Foucault, Michel. 1982. *The Archaeology of Knowledge: And the Discourse on Language*, New York: Vintage.

Fox, Nick J. 2016. "Health Sociology from Post-Structuralism to the New Materialisms." *Health* 20(1):62–74.

Fox, Renee. 1979. *Essays in Medical Sociology: Journeys into the Fields*. Piscataway, NJ: Transaction Publishers.

Freeman, Jo, and Victoria Johnson. 1999. *Waves of Protest: Social Movements since the Sixties*. Lanham, MD: Rowman & Littlefield.

Freidson, Eliot. 1988. *Profession of Medicine: A Study of the Sociology of Applied Knowledge*. Chicago: University of Chicago Press.

Freidson, Eliot. 1984. "The Changing Nature of Professional Control." *Annual Review of Sociology* 10(1):1–20.

Frickel, Scott, and Kelly Moore. 2006. *The New Political Sociology of Science: Institutions, Networks, and Power.* Madison: University of Wisconsin Press.

Friesen, Phoebe. 2018. "Educational Pelvic Exams on Anesthetized Women: Why Consent Matters." *Bioethics* 32(5):298–307.

Gimlin, Debra. 2007. "What Is 'Body Work'? A Review of the Literature." *Sociology Compass* 1(1):353–370.

Giuffre, Patti A., and Christine L. Williams. 2000. "Not Just Bodies: Strategies for Desexualizing the Physical Examination of Patients." *Gender & Society* 14(3):457–482.

Godkins, Thomas R., Daniel Duffy, Judith Greenwood, and William D. Stanhope. 1974. "Utilization of Simulated Patients to Teach the Routine Pelvic Examination." *Academic Medicine* 49(12):1174–1178.

Goldner, Melinda. 2004. "The Dynamic Interplay between Western Medicine and the Complementary and Alternative Medicine Movement: How Activists Perceive a Range of Responses from Physicians and Hospitals." *Sociology of Health & Illness* 26(6):710–736.

Gordon, Howard S., Richard L. Street Jr, Barbara F. Sharf, and Julianne Souchek. 2006. "Racial Differences in Doctors' Information-Giving and Patients' Participation." *Cancer* 107(6):1313–1320.

Gould, Deborah B. 2009. *Moving Politics: Emotion and ACT UP's Fight against AIDS.* Chicago: University of Chicago Press.

Goyal, Monika K., Nathan Kuppermann, Sean D. Cleary, Stephen J. Teach, and James M. Chamberlain. 2015. "Racial Disparities in Pain Management of Children with Appendicitis in Emergency Departments." *JAMA Pediatrics* 169(11):996–1002.

Grosz, Elizabeth A. 1994. *Volatile Bodies: Toward a Corporeal Feminism.* Bloomington: Indiana University Press.

Guarrasi, Ivana. 2015. "Residual Categories in Medical Simulation: The Role of Affect in the Performance of Disease." *Mind, Culture, and Activity* 22(2):112–128.

Guenther, Susan M., Douglas W. Laube, and Sandra Matthes. 1983. "Effectiveness of the Gynecology Teaching Associate in Teaching Pelvic Examination Skills." *Academic Medicine* 58(1):67–69.

Hafferty, Frederic W. 1988. "Cadaver Stories and the Emotional Socialization of Medical Students." *Journal of Health and Social Behavior* 29(4): 344–356.

Hafferty, Frederic W., and Brian Castellani. 2011. "Two Cultures: Two Ships: The Rise of a Professionalism Movement within Modern Medicine and Medical Sociology's Disappearance from the Professionalism Debate." Pp. 201–219 in *Handbook of the Sociology of Health, Illness, and Healing,* edited by Bernice A. Pescosolido, Jack K. Martin, Jane D. McLeod, and Anne Rogers. New York: Springer.

Hafferty, Frederic W., and Brian Castellani. 2009. "The Hidden Curriculum: A Theory of Medical Education." Pp. 29–49 in *Handbook of the Sociology of Medical Education,* edited by Caragh Brosnan and Bryan J. Turner. New York: Routledge.

Hall, Judith A., Susan A. Andrzejewski, and Jennelle E. Yopchick. 2009. "Psychosocial Correlates of Interpersonal Sensitivity: A Meta-Analysis." *Journal of Nonverbal Behavior* 33(3):149–180.

Halpern, Jodi. 2011. *From Detached Concern to Empathy: Humanizing Medical Practice.* New York: Oxford University Press.

Hammer, Gili. 2018. "'You Can Learn Merely by Listening to the Way a Patient Walks through the Door': The Transmission of Sensory Medical Knowledge." *Medical Anthropology Quarterly* 32(1):138–154.

Hansen, Helena, Joel Braslow, and Robert M. Rohrbaugh. 2018. "From Cultural to Structural Competency—Training Psychiatry Residents to Act on Social Determinants of Health and Institutional Racism." *JAMA Psychiatry* 75(2):117–118.

Harden, R. T. M., Mary Stevenson, W. Wilson Downie, and G. M. Wilson. 1975. "Assessment of Clinical Competence Using Objective Structured Examination." *British Medical Journal* 1(5955):447–451.

Harden, Ronald M., and F. A. Gleeson. 1979. "Assessment of Clinical Competence Using an Objective Structured Clinical Examination (OSCE)." *Medical Education* 13(1):39–54.

Hardt, Michael. 1999. "Affective Labor." *Boundary 2* 26(2):89–100.

Hardt, Michael, and Antonio Negri. 2001. *Empire.* Cambridge, MA: Harvard University Press.

Harris, Anna. 2016. "Listening-Touch, Affect and the Crafting of Medical Bodies through Percussion." *Body & Society* 22(1):31–61.

Harter, Lynn M., and Erika L. Kirby. 2004. "Socializing Medical Students in an Era of Managed Care: The Ideological Significance of Standardized and Virtual Patients." *Communication Studies* 55(1):48–67.

Hasle, Josie L., Delia S. Anderson, and Harold M. Szerlip. 1994. "Analysis of the Costs and Benefits of Using Standardized Patients to Help Teach Physical Diagnosis." *Academic Medicine: Journal of the Association of American Medical Colleges* 69(7):567–570.

Haug, Marie R. 1988. "A Re-Examination of the Hypothesis of Physician Deprofessionalization." *Milbank Quarterly* 66(2):48–56.

Hautz, Wolf E., Therese Schröder, Katja A. Dannenberg, Maren März, Henrike Hölzer, Olaf Ahlers, and Anke Thomas. 2017. "Shame in Medical Education: A Randomized Study of the Acquisition of Intimate Examination Skills and Its Effect on Subsequent Performance." *Teaching and Learning in Medicine* 29(2):196–206.

Helfer, Ray, and Joseph Hess. 1970. "An Experimental Model for Making Objective Measurements of Interviewing Skills." *Journal of Clinical Psychology* 26(3):327–331.

Henry-Tillman, Ronda, Linda A. Deloney, Mildred Savidge, C. James Graham, and V. Suzanne Klimberg. 2002. "The Medical Student as Patient Navigator as an Approach to Teaching Empathy." *American Journal of Surgery* 183(6):659–662.

Henslin, James M., and Mae A. Biggs. 1971. "Dramaturgical Desexualization: The Sociology of the Vaginal Examination." Pp. 243–272 in *Studies in the Sociology of Sex*, edited by James M. Henslin. New York: Appleton-Century-Crofts.

Hoang, Kimberly Kay. 2015. *Dealing in Desire: Asian Ascendancy, Western Decline, and the Hidden Currencies of Global Sex Work.* Berkeley: University of California Press.

Hochschild, Arlie Russell. 2012. *The Managed Heart: Commercialization of Human Feeling.* Berkeley: University of California Press.

Hodges, Brian. 2006. "Medical Education and the Maintenance of Incompetence." *Medical Teacher* 28(8):690–696.

Hoffman, Steve G. 2006. "How to Punch Someone and Stay Friends: An Inductive Theory of Simulation." *Sociological Theory* 24(2):170–193.

Holzberg, Billy. 2018. "The Multiple Lives of Affect: A Case Study of Commercial Surrogacy." *Body & Society* 24(4):32–57.

Howell, Mary C. 1974. "*What Medical Schools Teach about Women.*" *New England Journal of Medicine* 291:304–307.

Illouz, Eva. 2007. *Cold Intimacies: The Making of Emotional Capitalism.* Cambridge, UK: Polity.

Irby, David M., Molly Cooke, and Bridget C. O'Brien. 2010. "Calls for Reform of Medical Education by the Carnegie Foundation for the Advancement of Teaching: 1910 and 2010." *Academic Medicine* 85(2):220–227.

Irwin, W. G., R. McClelland, and A. H. G. Love. 1989. "Communication Skills Training for Medical Students: An Integrated Approach." *Medical Education* 23(4):387–394.

Jacques, Louis. 2003. "Use of Gynecology Teaching Models in the US." *British Medical Journal* 327:1389.

Janjua, Aisha, Tracy Roberts, Nicola Okeahialam, and T. Justin Clark. 2018. "Cost-Effective Analysis of Teaching Pelvic Examination Skills Using Gynaecology Teaching Associates (GTAs) Compared with Manikin Models (The CEAT Study)." *BMJ Open* 8(6):e015823.

Janjua, Aisha, P. Smith, J. Chu, N. Raut, S. Malick, I. Gallos, R. Singh, S. Irani, J. K. Gupta, and J. Parle. 2017. "The Effectiveness of Gynaecology Teaching Associates in Teaching Pelvic Examination to Medical Students: A Randomised Controlled Trial." *European Journal of Obstetrics & Gynecology and Reproductive Biology* 210:58–63.

Jay, Melanie, Adina Kalet, Tavinder Ark, Michelle McMacken, Mary Jo Messito, Regina Richter, Sheira Schlair, Scott Sherman, Sondra Zabar, and Colleen Gillespie. 2009. "Physicians' Attitudes about Obesity and Their Associations with Competency and Specialty: A Cross-Sectional Study." *BMC Health Services Research* 9(1):106–116.

Jenkins, Tania M. 2018. "Dual Autonomies, Divergent Approaches: How Stratification in Medical Education Shapes Approaches to Patient Care." *Journal of Health and Social Behavior* 59(2): 268–282.

Jewson, Nicholas D. 1976. "The Disappearance of the Sick-Man from Medical Cosmology, 1770–1870." *Sociology* 10(2):225–244.

Johnson, Gary H., Thomas C. Brown, Morton A. Stenchever, Harvey A. Gabert, A. Marsh Poulson, and James C. Warenski. 1975. "Teaching Pelvic Examination to Second-Year Medical Students Using Programmed Patients." *American Journal of Obstetrics and Gynecology* 121(5):714–717.

Johnson, Rachel L., Debra Roter, Neil R. Powe, and Lisa A. Cooper. 2004. "Patient Race/Ethnicity and Quality of Patient–Physician Communication during Medical Visits." *American Journal of Public Health* 94(12):2084–2090.

Joyce, Kelly Ann. 2008. *Magnetic Appeal: MRI and the Myth of Transparency*. Ithaca, NY: Cornell University Press.

Jupp, Eleanor, Jessica Pykett, and Fiona M. Smith. 2016. *Emotional States: Sites and Spaces of Affective Governance*. New York: Taylor & Francis.

Kang, Miliann. 2010. *The Managed Hand: Race, Gender, and the Body in Beauty Service Work*. Berkeley: University of California Press.

Kang, Miliann. 2003. "The Managed Hand: The Commercialization of Bodies and Emotions in Korean Immigrant–Owned Nail Salons." *Gender & Society* 17(6):820–839.

Kapsalis, Terri. 1997. *Public Privates: Performing Gynecology from Both Ends of the Speculum*. Durham, NC: Duke University Press.

Kassebaum, Donald G., and Robert H. Eaglen. 1999. "Shortcomings in the Evaluation of Students' Clinical Skills and Behaviors in Medical School." *Academic Medicine: Journal of the Association of American Medical Colleges* 74(7):842–849.

Kavinoky, Nadina R. 1954. "Premarital Medical Examination." *JAMA* 156(7):692–695.

Kendall, Patricia L., and George G. Reader. 1988. "Innovations in Medical Education of the 1950s Contrasted with Those of the 1970s and 1980s." *Journal of Health and Social Behavior* 29(4):279–293.

Kesti, Julie. 2010. "Plastic Pelvises Do Not Prepare Doctors for Real Ones." *Minnesota Daily*, February 17.

Khan, Kamran Z., Sankaranarayanan Ramachandran, Kathryn Gaunt, and Piyush Pushkar. 2013. "The Objective Structured Clinical Examination (OSCE): AMEE Guide No. 81. Part I: An Historical and Theoretical Perspective." *Medical Teacher* 35(9):e1437–e1446.

Klawiter, Maren. 2008. *The Biopolitics of Breast Cancer: Changing Cultures of Disease and Activism*. Minneapolis: University of Minnesota Press.

Kline, Wendy. 2010. *Bodies of Knowledge: Sexuality, Reproduction, and Women's Health in the Second Wave*. Chicago: University of Chicago Press.

Kretzschmar, Robert M. 1978. "Evolution of the Gynecology Teaching Associate: An Education Specialist." *American Journal of Obstetrics and Gynecology* 131(4):367–373.

Kuper, Ayelet, Mathieu Albert, and Brian David Hodges. 2010. "The Origins of the Field of Medical Education Research." *Academic Medicine* 85(8):1347–1353.

Kupfer, Joel M., and Edward U. Bond. 2012. "Patient Satisfaction and Patient-Centered Care: Necessary but Not Equal." *JAMA* 308(2):139–140.

Kuppers, Petra. 2008. "Remembering Anarcha: Objection in the Medical Archive." *Liminalities: A Journal of Performance Studies* 4(2):1–34.

Laine, Christine, and Frank Davidoff. 1996. "Patient-Centered Medicine: A Professional Evolution." *JAMA* 275(2):152–156.

Lakoff, Andrew. 2017. "A Fragile Assemblage: Mutant Bird Flu and the Limits of Risk Assessment." *Social Studies of Science* 47(3):376–397.

Larson, Eric B., and Xin Yao. 2005. "Clinical Empathy as Emotional Labor in the Patient-Physician Relationship." *JAMA* 293(9):1100–1106.

Latour, Bruno. 2004. "How to Talk about the Body? The Normative Dimension of Science Studies." *Body & Society* 10(2–3):205–229.

Lee, Robert. 1851. "On the Use of the Speculum in the Diagnosis and Treatment of Uterine Diseases." *Edinburgh Medical and Surgical Journal* 33(1):261–278.

Lee, Philip R., and Patricia E. Franks. 2010. "Diversity in US Medical Schools: Revitalizing Efforts to Increase Diversity in a Changing Context, 1960–2000s." Philip R. Lee Institute for Health Policy Studies. University of California, San Francisco, School of Medicine.

Lempp, Heidi. 2009. "Medical-School Culture." Pp. 85–102 in *Handbook of the Sociology of Medical Education*, edited by Caragh Brosnan and Bryan S. Turner. New York: Routledge.

Levinson, Wendy, Debra L. Roter, John P. Mullooly, Valerie T. Dull, and Richard M. Frankel. 1997. "Physician-Patient Communication: The Relationship with Malpractice Claims among Primary Care Physicians and Surgeons." *JAMA* 277(7):553–559.

Lewis, Carolyn Herbst. 2010. *Prescription for Heterosexuality*. Durham: University of North Carolina Press.

Lewis, Carolyn Herbst. 2005. "Waking Sleeping Beauty: The Premarital Pelvic Exam and Heterosexuality during the Cold War." *Journal of Women's History* 17(4):86–110.

Lewis, Sophie. 2016. "Gestational Labors: Care Politics and Surrogates' Struggle." Pp. 187–212 in *Intimate Economies*, edited by Susanne Hofmann and Adi Moreno. New York: Palgrave Macmillan US.

Light, Donald W. 1991. "Professionalism as a Countervailing Power." *Journal of Health Politics, Policy and Law* 16(3):499–506.

Linn, Lawrence S., Robert K. Oye, Dennis W. Cope, and M. Robin DiMatteo. 1986. "Use of Nonphysician Staff to Evaluate Humanistic Behavior of Internal Medicine Residents and Faculty Members." *Academic Medicine* 61(11):918–920.

Livingstone, Ronald A., and David N. Ostrow. 1978. "Professional Patient-Instructors in the Teaching of the Pelvic Examination." *American Journal of Obstetrics and Gynecology* 132(1):64–67.

Long, W. Newton. 1990. "The Pelvic Examination." Pp. 827–829 in *Clinical Methods: The History, Physical, and Laboratory Methods*, edited by H. Kenneth Walker, W. Dallas Hall, and J. Willis Hurst. Oxford, UK: Butterworth-Heinemann.

López, Iris Ofelia. 2008. *Matters of Choice: Puerto Rican Women's Struggle for Reproductive Freedom*. New Brunswick, NJ: Rutgers University Press.

Löwy, Ilana. 2010. "Cancer, Women, and Public Health: The History of Screening for Cervical Cancer." *História, Ciências, Saúde-Manguinhos* 17(1):53–67.

Luke, H. 2003. *Medical Education and Sociology of Medical Habitus: "It's Not about the Stethoscope!"* New York: Springer Science & Business Media.

MacFife, Bex. 2019. "The Not-So-Typical Patient: Gynecological Teaching Associates and the Struggle to Queer Medicine." PhD dissertation. San Francisco State University, San Francisco, CA.

Magee, Joni. 1975. "The Pelvic Examination: A View from the Other End of the Table." *Annals of Internal Medicine* 83(4):563–564.

Makoul, Gregory. 2001. "The SEGUE Framework for Teaching and Assessing Communication Skills." *Patient Education and Counseling* 45(1):23–34.

Mamo, Laura. 2007. *Queering Reproduction: Achieving Pregnancy in the Age of Technoscience*. Durham, NC: Duke University Press.

Mamo, Laura, and Jennifer Ruth Fosket. 2009. "Scripting the Body: Pharmaceuticals and the (Re)Making of Menstruation." *Signs: Journal of Women in Culture and Society* 34(4):925–949.

Mankekar, Purnima, and Akhil Gupta. 2016. "Intimate Encounters: Affective Labor in Call Centers." *Positions: East Asia Cultures Critique* 24(1):17–43.

Mann, Karen V. 2011. "Theoretical Perspectives in Medical Education: Past Experience and Future Possibilities." *Medical Education* 45(1):60–68.

Martin, Aryn, Natasha Myers, and Ana Viseu. 2015. "The Politics of Care in Technoscience." *Social Studies of Science* 45(5):625–641.

Martin, Emily. 2001. *The Woman in the Body: A Cultural Analysis of Reproduction*. Boston: Beacon Press.

Massumi, Brian. 2002. *Parables for the Virtual: Movement, Affect, Sensation*. Durham, NC: Duke University Press.

Matziou, Vasiliki, Efrosyni Vlahioti, Pantelis Perdikaris, Theodora Matziou, Efstathia Megapanou, and Konstantinos Petsios. 2014. "Physician and Nursing Perceptions Concerning Interprofessional Communication and Collaboration." *Journal of Interprofessional Care* 28(6):526–533.

Maynard, Alan, and Alan Williams. 2018. "Privatisation and the National Health Service." Pp. 95–110 in *Privatisation and the Welfare State*, edited by Julian Le Grand and Ray Robinson. New York: Routledge.

McCabe, Katharine. 2016. "Mothercraft: Birth Work and the Making of Neoliberal Mothers." *Social Science & Medicine* 162:177–184.

McGregor, Deborah Kuhn. 1998. *From Midwives to Medicine: The Birth of American Gynecology*. New Brunswick, NJ: Rutgers University Press.

McKinlay, John B., and Joan Arches. 1985. "Towards the Proletarianization of Physicians." *International Journal of Health Services* 15(2):161–195.

McNay, Lois. 1999. "Gender, Habitus and the Field: Pierre Bourdieu and the Limits of Reflexivity." *Theory, Culture & Society* 16(1):95–117.

Mears, Ashley. 2014. "Aesthetic Labor for the Sociologies of Work, Gender, and Beauty." *Sociology Compass* 8(12):1330–1343.

Merleau-Ponty, Maurice. 2013. *Phenomenology of Perception*. New York: Routledge.

Metzl, Jonathan, and Anna Kirkland. 2010. *Against Health: How Health Became the New Morality*. New York: New York University Press.

Miller, George E. 1994. "The Clinical Skills Assessment Alliance." *Academic Medicine* 69(4): 285–287.

Miller, George E. 1990. "The Assessment of Clinical Skills/Competence/Performance." *Academic Medicine* 65(9):S63–S67.

Miller, George E. 1980. *Educating Medical Teachers*. Cambridge, MA: Harvard University Press.

Mol, Annemarie, and John Law. 2004. "Embodied Action, Enacted Bodies: The Example of Hypoglycaemia." *Body & Society* 10(2–3):43–62.

Morgen, Sandra. 2002. *Into Our Own Hands: The Women's Health Movement in the United States, 1969–1990*. New Brunswick, NJ: Rutgers University Press.

Moseby, Kevin M. 2017. "Two Regimes of HIV/AIDS: The MMWR and the Socio-Political Construction of HIV/AIDS as a 'Black Disease.'" *Sociology of Health & Illness* 39(7):1068–1082.

Murphy, Michelle. 2015. "Unsettling Care: Troubling Transnational Itineraries of Care in Feminist Health Practices." *Social Studies of Science* 45(5):717–737.

Murphy, Michelle. 2012. *Seizing the Means of Reproduction: Entanglements of Feminism, Health, and Technoscience*. Durham, NC: Duke University Press.

Murphy, Michelle. 2004. "Immodest Witnessing: The Epistemology of Vaginal Self-Examination in the US Feminist Self-Help Movement." *Feminist Studies* 30(1):115–147.

Myers, Natasha. 2012. "Dance Your PhD: Embodied Animations, Body Experiments, and the Affective Entanglements of Life Science Research." *Body & Society* 18(1):151–189.

National Center for Health Statistics. 2016. "National Ambulatory Medical Care Survey: 2016 National Summary Tables." https://www.cdc.gov.

National Public Radio. 2018. "661: But That's What Happened." *This American Life*, November 9. https://www.thisamericanlife.org.

Nelson, Alondra. 2016. *The Social Life of DNA: Race, Reparations, and Reconciliation after the Genome*. Boston: Beacon Press.

Nelson, Alondra. 2011. *Body and Soul: The Black Panther Party and the Fight against Medical Discrimination*. Minneapolis: University of Minnesota Press.

Nelson, Lewis H. 1978. "Use of Professional Patients in Teaching Pelvic Examinations." *Obstetrics and Gynecology* 52(5):630–633.

Norsigian, Judy. 1975. "Training the Docs." *Healthright* Winter.

Northup, Diana E. 1984. "Humanizing the Business of Medicine: The Use of Simulated Patients to Train Medical Students." in *Developments in Business Simulation and Experiential Learning: Proceedings of the Annual Association for Business Simulation and Experiential Learning Conference* 11:232–234.

Nutter, Donald, and Michael Whitcomb. 2001. "The AAMC Project on the Clinical Education of Medical Students." Washington, DC: American Association of Medical Colleges.

Oeffinger, Kevin C., Elizabeth T. H. Fontham, Ruth Etzioni, Abbe Herzig, James S. Michaelson, Ya-Chen Tina Shih, Louise C. Walter, Timothy R. Church, Christopher R. Flowers, and Samuel J. LaMonte. 2015. "Breast Cancer Screening for Women at Average Risk: 2015 Guideline Update from the American Cancer Society." *JAMA* 314(15):1599–1614.

Okwerekwu, Jennifer Adaeze. 2016. "Medical Students Demand an End to Pricey Licensing Exam." *STAT*, March 11.

Olsen, Lauren D. 2019. "The Conscripted Curriculum and the Reproduction of Racial Inequalities in Contemporary US Medical Education." *Journal of Health and Social Behavior* 60(1):55–68.

Ong, Aihwa, and Stephen Collier. 2008. *Global Assemblages:* Technology, Politics, and Ethics as Anthropological Problems. New York: Wiley.

Orr, Jackie. 2006. *Panic Diaries: A Genealogy of Panic Disorder.* Durham, NC: Duke University Press.

Owens, Deirdre Cooper. 2017. *Medical Bondage: Race, Gender, and the Origins of American Gynecology.* Athens: University of Georgia Press.

Pande, Amrita. 2010. "Commercial Surrogacy in India: Manufacturing a Perfect Mother-Worker." *Signs: Journal of Women in Culture and Society* 35(4):969–992.

Patel, R. S., C. Tarrant, S. Bonas, and R. L. Shaw. 2015. "Medical Students' Personal Experience of High-Stakes Failure: Case Studies Using Interpretative Phenomenological Analysis." *BMC Medical Education* 15(1):86–94.

Paterson, Mark. 2007. *The Senses of Touch: Haptics, Affects and Technologies.* Oxford, UK: Berg Publishers.

Patrício, Madalena Folque, Miguel Julião, Filipa Fareleira, and António Vaz Carneiro. 2013. "Is the OSCE a Feasible Tool to Assess Competencies in Undergraduate Medical Education?" *Medical Teacher* 35(6):503–514.

Pedersen, Reidar. 2010. "Empathy Development in Medical Education–A Critical Review." *Medical Teacher* 32(7):593–600.

Perlmutter, J. F., and E. A. Friedman. 1974. "Use of a Live Mannequin for Teaching Physical Diagnosis in Gynecology." *Journal of Reproductive Medicine* 12(4):163–164.

Pho, Kevin. 2010. "Pelvic Exam Simulators Do Medical Students a Disservice." Blog. KevinMD.com. www.kevinmd.com.

Piper, Llewellyn E., and Erin Tallman. 2016. "Hospital Consumer Assessment of Healthcare Providers and Systems: An Ethical Leadership Dilemma to Satisfy Patients." *Health Care Manager* 35(2):151–155.

Pitts-Taylor, Victoria. 2016. *Mattering: Feminism, Science, and Materialism.* New York: New York University Press.

Plauché, Warren C., and Wendy Baugniet-Nebrija. 1985. "Students' and Physicians' Evaluations of Gynecologic Teaching Associate Program." *Journal of Medical Education* 60(11)870–875.

Posner, Glenn D. 2015. "The Quandary of the Sacred Vagina: Exploring the Value of Gynaecological Teaching Associates." *Medical Education* 49(12):1179–1180.

Potter, Sharyn J., and John B. McKinlay. 2005. "From a Relationship to Encounter: An Examination of Longitudinal and Lateral Dimensions in the Doctor-Patient Relationship." *Social Science & Medicine* 61(2):465–479.

Prentice, Rachel. 2013. *Bodies in Formation: An Ethnography of Anatomy and Surgery Education.* Durham, NC: Duke University Press.

Price, Tristan, Nick Lynn, Lee Coombes, Martin Roberts, Tom Gale, Sam Regan de Bere, and Julian Archer. 2018. "The International Landscape of Medical Licensing

Examinations: A Typology Derived from a Systematic Review." *International Journal of Health Policy and Management* 7(9):782–790.

Puar, Jasbir. 2007. *Terrorist Assemblages: Homonationalism in Queer Times.* Durham, NC: Duke University Press.

Rangel, Jaime C., Carrie Cartmill, Ayelet Kuper, Maria A. Martimianakis, and Cynthia R. Whitehead. 2016. "Setting the Standard: Medical Education's First 50 Years." *Medical Education* 50(1):24–35.

Reeder, Leo G. 1972. "The Patient-Client as a Consumer: Some Observations on the Changing Professional-Client Relationship." *Journal of Health and Social Behavior* 13(4):406–412.

Regenstein, Marsha, Jennifer Trott, Alanna Williamson, and Joanna Theiss. 2018. "Addressing Social Determinants of Health through Medical-Legal Partnerships." *Health Affairs* 37(3):378–385.

Reich, Adam. 2012. "Disciplined Doctors: The Electronic Medical Record and Physicians' Changing Relationship to Medical Knowledge." *Social Science & Medicine* 74(7):1021–1028.

Ricci, James V. 1949. *The Development of Gynaecological Surgery and Instruments.* Philadelphia: The Blakiston Company.

Richard, Analiese, and Daromir Rudnyckyj. 2009. "Economies of Affect." *Journal of the Royal Anthropological Institute* 15(1):57–77.

Ringrose, Jessica, and Emma Renold. 2014. "'F** k Rape!' Exploring Affective Intensities in a Feminist Research Assemblage." *Qualitative Inquiry* 20(6):772–780.

Rizwan, Muhammad, Nicole J. Rosson, Sean Tackett, and Heitham T. Hassoun. n.d. "Globalization of Medical Education: Current Trends and Opportunities for Medical Students." *Journal of Medical Education and Training* 2(1): 35–41.

Roberts, Dorothy. 2015. "Reproductive Justice, Not Just Rights." *Dissent Magazine.* https://www.dissentmagazine.org.

Roberts, Dorothy E. 1999. *Killing the Black Body: Race, Reproduction, and the Meaning of Liberty.* New York: Vintage Books.

Rollnick, Stephen, William R. Miller, and Christopher Butler. 2008. *Motivational Interviewing in Health Care: Helping Patients Change Behavior.* New York: Guilford Press.

Rose, Nikolas. 2009. *The Politics of Life Itself: Biomedicine, Power, and Subjectivity in the Twenty-First Century.* Princeton, NJ: Princeton University Press.

Rose, Nikolas. 1998. *Inventing Our Selves: Psychology, Power, and Personhood.* New York: Cambridge University Press.

Rose, Nikolas. 1993. "Government, Authority and Expertise in Advanced Liberalism." *Economy and Society* 22(3):283–299.

Rosinski, Edwin F. 1988. *The Society of Directors of Research in Medical Education: A Brief History.* Office of Medical Education, University of California, San Francisco.

Ross, Steven E. 1962. "Programmed Instruction and Medical Education." *JAMA* 182(9):938–939.

Rothstein, William G. 1987. *American Medical Schools and the Practice of Medicine: A History*. New York: Oxford University Press.

Ruzek, Sheryl Burt, and Julie Becker. 1999. "The Women's Health Movement in the United States: From Grass-Roots Activism to Professional Agendas." *JAMWA* 54(1):4–8.

Sabin, Janice A., Maddalena Marini, and Brian A. Nosek. 2012. "Implicit and Explicit Anti-Fat Bias among a Large Sample of Medical Doctors by BMI, Race/Ethnicity and Gender." *PloS One* 7(11):e48448.

Salmon, J. Warren. 1985. "Profit and Health Care: Trends in Corporatization and Proprietization." *International Journal of Health Services* 15(3):395–418.

Sanson-Fisher, R., Susan Fairbairn, and P. Maguire. 1981. "Teaching Skills in Communication to Medical Students—A Critical Review of the Methodology." *Medical Education* 15(1):33–37.

Sarmasoglu, Senay, Leyla Dinc, Melih Elcin, Gul Hatice Tarakcioglu Celik, and Isle Polonko. 2016. "Success of the First Gynecological Teaching Associate Program in Turkey." *Clinical Simulation in Nursing* 12(8):305–312.

Saslow, George. 1948. "An Experiment with Comprehensive Medicine." *Psychosomatic Medicine* 10(3):165–175.

Schuller, Kyla. 2017. *The Biopolitics of Feeling: Race, Sex, and Science in the Nineteenth Century*. Durham, NC: Duke University Press.

Schwartz, Marlene B., Heather O'Neal Chambliss, Kelly D. Brownell, Steven N. Blair, and Charles Billington. 2003. "Weight Bias among Health Professionals Specializing in Obesity." *Obesity Research* 11(9):1033–1039.

Seegal, David, and Arthur R. Wertheim. 1962. "On the Failure to Supervise Students Performance of Complete Physical Examinations." *JAMA* 180(6):476–477.

Shain, Rochelle N., S. H. Crouch, and P. C. Weinberg. 1982. "Evaluation of the Gynecology Teaching Associate versus Pelvic Model Approach to Teaching Pelvic Examination." *Academic Medicine* 57(8):646–648.

Shanafelt, Tait D., Lotte N. Dyrbye, and Colin P. West. 2017. "Addressing Physician Burnout: The Way Forward." *JAMA* 317(9):901–902.

Shim, Janet K. 2010. "Cultural Health Capital: A Theoretical Approach to Understanding Health Care Interactions and the Dynamics of Unequal Treatment." *Journal of Health and Social Behavior* 51(1):1–15.

Silverman, David, and Michael Bloor. 1990. "Patient Centred Medicine: Some Sociological Observations on Its Constitution, Penetration, and Cultural Assonance." *Advances in Medical Sociology* 1:3–25.

Sinclair, Simon. 1997. *Making Doctors: An Institutional Apprenticeship*. Oxford, UK: Berg.

Smith, Allen C., and Sherryl Kleinman. 1989. "Managing Emotions in Medical School: Students' Contacts with the Living and the Dead." *Social Psychology Quarterly* 52(1):56–69.

Smith, Molly, and Juno Mac. 2018. *Revolting Prostitutes: The Fight for Sex Workers' Rights*. New York: Verso.

Smith, Paul P., Shelina Choudhury, and T. Justin Clark. 2015. "The Effectiveness of Gynaecological Teaching Associates in Teaching Pelvic Examination: A Systematic Review and Meta-Analysis." *Medical Education* 49(12):1197–1206.

Snorton, C. Riley. 2017. *Black on Both Sides: A Racial History of Trans Identity*. Minneapolis: University of Minnesota Press.

Sointu, Eeva. 2017. "'Good' Patient/'Bad' Patient: Clinical Learning and the Entrenching of Inequality." *Sociology of Health & Illness* 39(1):63–77.

Starr, Paul. 1982. *The Social Transformation of American Medicine*. New York: Basic Books.

Stern, Scott W. 2018. *The Trials of Nina McCall: Sex, Surveillance, and the Decades-Long Government Plan to Imprison "Promiscuous" Women*. Boston: Beacon Press.

Stewart, Felicia H., Cynthia C. Harper, Charlotte E. Ellertson, David A. Grimes, George F. Sawaya, and James Trussell. 2001. "Clinical Breast and Pelvic Examination Requirements for Hormonal Contraception: Current Practice vs. Evidence." *JAMA* 285(17):2232–2239.

Stewart, Moira A., Judith Belle Brown, W. Wayne Weston, Ian R. McWhinney, Carol L. McWilliam, and Thomas R. Freeman. 2014. *Patient-Centered Medicine, Third Edition: Transforming the Clinical Method*. London: Radcliff Publishing.

Stillman, Paula L., David R. Brown, Doris L. Redfield, and Darrell L. Sabers. 1977. "Construct Validation of the Arizona Clinical Interview Rating Scale." *Educational and Psychological Measurement* 37(4):1031–1038.

Stillman, Paula L., Mary B. Regan, Mary Philbin, and Heather-Lyn Haley. 1990a. "Results of a Survey on the Use of Standardized Patients to Teach and Evaluate Clinical Skills." *Academic Medicine* 65(5):288–292.

Stillman, Paula L., Mary B. Regan, David B. Swanson, Susan Case, J. McCahan, J. Feinblatt, S. R. Smith, J. Willms, and D. V. Nelson. 1990b. "An Assessment of the Clinical Skills of Fourth-Year Students at Four New England Medical Schools." *Academic Medicine* 65(5):320–326.

Stillman, Paula L., and David B. Swanson. 1987. "Ensuring the Clinical Competence of Medical School Graduates through Standardized Patients." *Archives of Internal Medicine* 147(6):1049–1052.

Stroumsa, Daphna, Deirdre A. Shires, Caroline R. Richardson, Kim D. Jaffee, and Michael R. Woodford. 2019. "Transphobia Rather than Education Predicts Provider Knowledge of Transgender Health Care." *Medical Education* 53(4):398–407.

Swanson, David B., and Trudie E. Roberts. 2016. "Trends in National Licensing Examinations in Medicine." *Medical Education* 50(1):101–114.

Sweet, Paige L. 2018. "The Paradox of Legibility: Domestic Violence and Institutional Survivorhood." *Social Problems* 66(3):411–427.

Taylor, Chloë. 2011. "Biopower." Pp. 41–54 in *Michel Foucault: Key Concepts*, edited by Dianna Taylor. Durham, UK: Acumen.

Taylor, Daniel R., Bruce A. Bernstein, Eileen Carroll, Elizabeth Oquendo, Linda Peyton, and Lee M. Pachter. 2015. "Keeping the Heat on for Children's Health: A Successful Medical-Legal Partnership Initiative to Prevent Utility Shutoffs in Vulnerable Children." *Journal of Health Care for the Poor and Underserved* 26(3):676–685.

Teachman, Bethany A. and Kelly D. Brownell. 2001. "Implicit Anti-Fat Bias among Health Professionals: Is Anyone Immune?" *International Journal of Obesity* 25(10):1525–1531.

Teherani, Arianne, Karen E. Hauer, and Patricia O'Sullivan. 2008. "Can Simulations Measure Empathy? Considerations on How to Assess Behavioral Empathy via Simulations." *Patient Education and Counseling* 71(2):148–152.

Tekian, Ara. 2014. "Doctoral Programs in Health Professions Education." *Medical Teacher* 36(1):73–81.

Tekian, Ara, and Ilene Harris. 2012. "Preparing Health Professions Education Leaders Worldwide: A Description of Masters-Level Programs." *Medical Teacher* 34(1):52–58.

Thomas, Jan E., and Mary K. Zimmerman. 2007. "Feminism and Profit in American Hospitals: The Corporate Construction of Women's Health Centers." *Gender & Society* 21(3):359–383.

Thompson, Charis. 2005. *Making Parents: The Ontological Choreography of Reproductive Technologies*. Cambridge, MA: MIT Press.

Timmermans, Stefan. 2011. "The Joy of Science: Finding Success in a 'Failed' Randomized Clinical Trial." *Science, Technology, & Human Values* 36(4):549–572.

Timmermans, Stefan, and Alison Angell. 2001. "Evidence-Based Medicine, Clinical Uncertainty, and Learning to Doctor." *Journal of Health and Social Behavior* 42(4):342–359.

Timmermans, Stefan, and Marc Berg. 2010. *The Gold Standard: The Challenge of Evidence-Based Medicine and Standardization in Health Care*. Philadelphia: Temple University Press.

Timmermans, Stefan, and Marc Berg. 1997. "Standardization in Action: Achieving Local Universality through Medical Protocols." *Social Studies of Science* 27(2):273–305.

Timmermans, Stefan, and Hyeyoung Oh. 2010. "The Continued Social Transformation of the Medical Profession." *Journal of Health and Social Behavior* 51(1 Suppl):S94–S106.

Tomes, Nancy. 2016. *Remaking the American Patient: How Madison Avenue and Modern Medicine Turned Patients into Consumers*. Durham: University of North Carolina Press.

Tsai, Jennifer. 2019. "Medical Students Regularly Practice Pelvic Exams on Unconscious Patients. Should They?" *ELLE*, June. https://www.elle.com.

Turner, Bryan S. 1997. "From Governmentality to Risk." Pp. ix–xxi in *Foucault, Health and Medicine, edited by Robin Bunton and Alan Petersen. London: Routledge.

Turner, Bryan S. 1995. *Medical Power and Social Knowledge*. New York: Sage.

Twigg, Julia. 2000. "Carework as a Form of Bodywork." *Ageing & Society* 20(4):389–411.

Ubel, Peter A., Christopher Jepson, and Ari Silver-Isenstadt. 2003. "Don't Ask, Don't Tell: A Change in Medical Student Attitudes after Obstetrics/Gynecology

Clerkships toward Seeking Consent for Pelvic Examinations on an Anesthetized Patient." *American Journal of Obstetrics and Gynecology* 188(2):575–579.

Underman, Kelly. 2011. "'It's the Knowledge That Puts You in Control': The Embodied Labor of Gynecological Educators." *Gender & Society* 25(4):431–450.

Underman, Kelly, Danielle Giffort, Abbas Hyderi, and Laura E. Hirshfield. 2016. *Transgender Health: A Standardized Patient Case for Advanced Clerkship Students.* MedEdPORTAL Publications. https://www.mededportal.org/.

Underman, Kelly, and Laura E. Hirshfield. 2016. "Detached Concern?: Emotional Socialization in Twenty-First Century Medical Education." *Social Science & Medicine* 160:94–101.

United States Medical Licensing Examination. n.d. "Performance Data." https://www.usmle.org (retrieved August 6, 2019).

Vinson, Alexandra H. 2019. "Surgical Identity Play: The Anatomy Lab Revisited." *Symbolic Interaction.* https://doi.org/10.1002/symb.465.

Vinson, Alexandra H. 2016. "'Constrained Collaboration': Patient Empowerment Discourse as Resource for Countervailing Power." *Sociology of Health & Illness* 38(8):1364–1378.

Vinson, Alexandra H., and Kelly Underman. 2020. "Clinical Empathy as Emotional Labour in Medical Education and Medical Work." https://doi.org/10.1016/j.socscimed.2020.112904.

Vontver, Louis, David Irby, Phillip Rakestraw, Mark Haddock, Edward Prince, and Morton Stenchever. 1980. "The Effects of Two Methods of Pelvic Examination Instruction on Student Performance and Anxiety." *Journal of Medical Education* 55(9):778–785.

Vora, Kalindi. 2010. "The Transmission of Care." Pp. 33–48 in *Intimate Labors: Cultures, Technologies, and the Politics of Care,* edited by Eileen Boris and Rhacel Salazar Parreñas. Palo Alto, CA: Stanford University Press.

Wacquant, Loïc. 2014a. "Homines in Extremis: What Fighting Scholars Teach Us about Habitus." *Body & Society* 20(2):3–17.

Wacquant, Loïc. 2014b. "Putting Habitus in Its Place: Rejoinder to the Symposium." *Body & Society* 20(2):118–139.

Wacquant, Loïc. 2004. *Body & Soul.* Oxford, UK: Oxford University Press.

Wailoo, Keith, Alondra Nelson, and Catherine Lee. 2012. *Genetics and the Unsettled Past: The Collision of DNA, Race, and History.* New Brunswick, NJ: Rutgers University Press.

Waldby, Catherine. 2002. "Stem Cells, Tissue Cultures and the Production of Biovalue." *Health: An Interdisciplinary Journal for the Social Study of Health, Illness and Medicine* 6(3):305–323.

Wallace, Peggy. 1997. "Following the Threads of an Innovation: The History of Standardized Patients in Medical Education." *Caduceus* 13(2):5–28.

Washington, Harriet A. 2006. *Medical Apartheid: The Dark History of Medical Experimentation on Black Americans from Colonial Times to the Present.* New York: Doubleday.

Wear, Delese, and Joseph D. Varley. 2008. "Rituals of Verification: The Role of Simulation in Developing and Evaluating Empathic Communication." *Patient Education and Counseling* 71(2):153–156.

Weeks, Kathi. 2011. *The Problem with Work: Feminism, Marxism, Antiwork Politics, and Postwork Imaginaries*. Durham, NC: Duke University Press.

Weeks, Kathi. 2007. "Life within and against Work: Affective Labor, Feminist Critique, and Post-Fordist Politics." *Ephemera: Theory and Politics in Organization* 7(1):233–249.

Weiner, Saul, and Alan Schwartz. 2015. *Listening for What Matters: Avoiding Contextual Errors in Health Care*. New York: Oxford University Press.

Weiss, Kay. 1975. "What Medical Students Learn about Women." *Off Our Backs* 5(4):24–25.

West, Colin P., Liselotte N. Dyrbye, Patricia J. Erwin, and Tait D. Shanafelt. 2016. "Interventions to Prevent and Reduce Physician Burnout: A Systematic Review and Meta-Analysis." *The Lancet* 388(10057):2272–2281.

West, Colin P., Liselotte N. Dyrbye, and Tait D. Shanafelt. 2018. "Physician Burnout: Contributors, Consequences and Solutions." *Journal of Internal Medicine* 283(6):516–529.

West, Colin P., Tait D. Shanafelt, and Joseph C. Kolars. 2011. "Quality of Life, Burnout, Educational Debt, and Medical Knowledge among Internal Medicine Residents." *JAMA* 306(9):952–960.

Westbrook, Kevin W., Emin Babakus, and Cori Cohen Grant. 2014. "Measuring Patient-Perceived Hospital Service Quality: Validity and Managerial Usefulness of HCAHPS Scales." *Health Marketing Quarterly* 31(2):97–114.

Williams, Gareth. 1984. "The Genesis of Chronic Illness: Narrative Re-Construction." *Sociology of Health & Illness* 6(2):175–200.

Wilson, Robin Fretwell, and Anthony Michael Kreis. 2018. "#JustAsk: Stop Treating Unconscious Female Patients like Cadavers." *Chicago Tribune*, November 29.

Winefield, Helen R. 1982. "Subjective and Objective Outcomes of Communication Skills Training in First Year." *Medical Education* 16(4):192–196.

Wolfberg, Adam J. 2007. "The Patient as Ally—Learning the Pelvic Examination." *New England Journal of Medicine* 356(9):889–890.

Wolkowitz, Carol. 2006. *Bodies at Work*. New York: Sage.

Women's Community Health Center, Inc. 1976. "Experiences of a Pelvic Teaching Group." *Women & Health* 1(4):19–23.

Women's Community Health Center, Inc. 1976. "How to Do a Pelvic Examination." Personal communication.

Young, Katharine Galloway. 1997. *Presence in the Flesh: The Body in Medicine*. Cambridge, MA: Harvard University Press.

Zelizer, Viviana. 2010. "Caring Everywhere." Pp. 267–279 in *Intimate Labors: Cultures, Technologies, and the Politics of Care*, edited by Eileen Boris and Rhacel Salazar Parreñas. Palo Alto, CA: Stanford University Press.

Zelizer, Viviana. 2005. *The Purchase of Intimacy*. Princeton, NJ: Princeton University Press.

Zheng, Robin. 2018. "Precarity Is a Feminist Issue: Gender and Contingent Labor in the Academy." *Hypatia* 33(2):235–255.

Zimmerman, Mary K. 1987. "The Women's Health Movement: A Critique of Medical Enterprise and the Position of Women." Pp. 442–472 in *Analyzing Gender: A Handbook of Social Science Research*, edited by Beth B. Hess and Myra Marx Ferree. Thousand Oaks, CA: SAGE.

Ziv, Amitai, Paul Root Wolpe, Stephen D. Small, and Shimon Glick. 2003. "Simulation-Based Medical Education: An Ethical Imperative." *Academic Medicine* 78(8):783–788.

INDEX

abortion, 33, 39, 50

affect: and capitalism, 202–9; circulation of, 16, 164; definition, 3–4, 6, 15–16, 79, 205, 239n17; and emotion, 16, 142, 177, 205; and language, 55, 80–81, 144, 160–62; management of, 53, 67; regimes of, 18–19, 65, 113, 138–39, 169, 175, 184, 195, 198; technologies of, 19–22, 57, 60–61, 70, 78, 80–81, 85, 112, 116, 130, 167, 180, 195 189, 203–5, 209, 211–12, 222, 261. *See also* biopower; body/bodies: sensation of; habitus, medical

affective capacities, 4, 7, 10–11, 19, 28, 60–61, 79, 96, 146, 175, 181, 193, 196, 204–5, 208–9, 240n23

affective disposition, 116, 118, 120, 132, 138, 142, 193, 204

affective economies, 11, 17, 32, 52–53, 60–62, 102–6, 109, 111, 201, 206–7, 209, 213

affective governance, 17–20, 21–22, 57, 78, 84, 97, 140, 170, 175, 196, 198, 202–3, 210–11, 240n23

affective labor. See labor

affective resonance, 130, 135–38

affective ties, 97, 170, 204

affective turn in clinical medicine, 15–18, 240n23

agency, 33, 153–54, 206, 252n6

Ahmed, Sara, 17, 102, 240n23

anatomy lab, 1–2, 19, 118, 120

anatomy, normal, 43–44

anesthesia, patients under, 5, 29, 31, 199, 204, 242n10, 247n3, 255n4. *See also* pelvic exam

anonymous vagina. *See* vagina

anxiety, 2, 4, 14–15, 41, 46–47, 50, 52, 54, 71, 73–74, 85, 93, 97, 108, 115, 127, 131, 159–60, 184, 187. *See also* emotion/emotions

assemblage, 27, 38, 42, 145, 164–65, 205, 219, 227, 241n2, 241n3, 254n14. *See also* body/bodies

assessment, 60, 58, 64–65, 67, 69, 73–77, 83, 175, 179, 251n8; Likert scale, 74–75. *See also* clinical skills

Association of American Medical Colleges (AAMC), 7–8, 40, 69, 76, 221, 245n7, 245n8

attention, 22, 27, 70, 76, 85, 90, 97, 102, 109, 142–43, 149–52, 156–60, 165, 193

attentiveness, 21, 26, 68, 83–85, 94, 96, 99, 101

authenticity and artificiality, 130–36. *See also* simulation

authority, intimate, 78, 90–94, 97, 107–8, 111

authority, of physicians, 7, 43–44, 55, 62, 57, 65, 92, 203, 238n7, 240n1. *See also* professional dominance

Barad, Karen, 145, 252n6, 252n7, 253n9

Beckmann, Charles R. B., 41–45, 47, 52, 62, 66

bimanual exam. *See* pelvic exam

biomedicalization, 12, 20, 54, 190, 203, 208

biomedicine, 12, 15, 18, 20, 26, 34–35, 38, 41–44, 47, 54, 57, 65, 116, 130, 150, 170–79, 190, 192–95, 197, 223, 228

ABOUT THE AUTHOR

Kelly Underman is an Assistant Professor in the Department of Sociology at Drexel University.